Having Children
After Cancer

Having Children After Cancer

How to Make Informed Choices
Before and After Treatment and
Build the Family of Your Dreams

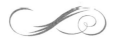

By Gina M. Shaw

Foreword by Hope S. Rugo, MD,
UCSF Comprehensive Cancer Center

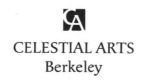

CELESTIAL ARTS
Berkeley

Published in the United States by Celestial Arts, an imprint of the Crown Publishing Group, a division of Random House, Inc., New York.
www.crownpublishing.com
www.tenspeed.com

Celestial Arts and the Celestial Arts colophon are registered trademarks of Random House, Inc.

Front cover photograph copyright © iStockphoto/Floortje

Library of Congress Cataloging-in-Publication Data
Shaw, Gina M.
  Having children after cancer : how to make informed choices before and after treatment and build the family of your dreams / by Gina M. Shaw.
     p. cm.
  Includes bibliographical references and index.
  Summary: "The first book to address fertility and cancer in a comprehensive, prescriptive way, explaining which cancers and treatments affect fertility and presenting a wide range of family-building options"—Provided by publisher.
  1. Infertility—Complications—Treatment—Popular works. 2. Cancer—Complications—Treatment—Popular works. I. Title.
  RC889.S49 2011
  616.99'4—dc22

                                                        2010028416

ISBN 978-1-58761-054-7

Printed in the United States of America on recycled paper (30% PCW)

Design by Chloe Rawlins

10 9 8 7 6 5 4 3 2 1

First Edition

Dedication

THIS BOOK IS LOVINGLY DEDICATED to two women who made it possible and who should have lived to see it published.

To the extraordinary Jeanne Petrek, MD, my breast surgeon at Memorial Sloan-Kettering Cancer Center in New York. She turned my cancer journey around from a train wreck to a narrative of survival, gave me confidence that I would survive and thrive, and helped make it possible for us to adopt our daughter.

Most important, to my mother, Dorothy Shaw. She taught me everything I needed to know in life—most especially, how to love and how to be a mother. Whenever I face a parenting challenge, I try to think "WWMD"—What Would Mom Do? I wish she could be here to see this book, but even more, to be the grandma she always wanted to be. I miss her every day. I love you, Mom.

I also dedicate this book to my amazing husband, Evan, and my three incredible kids, Annika, Adrian, and Katia. I'm so happy to wake up to you all (even in the predawn hours) every day.

Contents

Acknowledgments

THIS BOOK WOULD NOT HAVE been possible without the generous insights and expertise of the medical professionals, social workers, and other experts who took the time to share their experience with me. I am grateful to all the specialists interviewed for this book, especially the extraordinary staff at the Oncofertility Consortium at Northwestern University's Feinberg School of Medicine, who allowed me to spend time with them learning more about their groundbreaking work. Special thanks are also due to Lindsay Nohr Beck of Fertile Hope, who not only shared her own story but provided unique insights on the field of cancer, fertility, pregnancy, and parenting.

But even more than the professionals and experts, I owe thanks to the many families who took time to share their personal stories with me. Every family's journey through cancer to parenthood is a different one, yet in so many ways they are at heart the same: people who have fought one battle, to survive, and then had to wage yet another, to become parents—two things that most people take for granted. I can't thank you all enough for being willing to reach out to other families like yours through this book.

Special thanks are also due to my heroic husband, Evan, and three amazing kids, Annika, Adrian, and Katia; to my dad, Ronald

Shaw, who's always believed in me; to Annika's extraordinary birth mom, Kim, who gave us the joy of becoming parents for the first time; to my wonderful agent, Maria Massie of Lippincott Massie McQuilkin; and to the great cadre of friends who've cheered me on for the past several years as I worked to make the dream of this book a reality—especially Mark Rotella, who made that first connection!

Foreword

I FACED THE YOUNG WOMAN sitting in my office and discussed treatment options for her early-stage breast cancer, treatment necessary to give her the best chance of preventing recurrence. She faced the news of the recommendation for chemotherapy bravely. We then talked about the side effects of treatment, including the fact that her fertility could be adversely affected. She was incredulous that the treatment given to save her life could also change it so irrevocably, and was relieved to know that back-up plans were possible. We planned for her to meet with our fertility expert that same day, to learn about options for freezing eggs or embryos. Just having options and retaining some control over her future allowed this woman to move forward with treatment and all its challenges with a lifted spirit.

I am delighted to write the foreword to this groundbreaking book, *Having Children After Cancer*. As a breast cancer oncologist at the University of California San Francisco's Comprehensive Cancer Center, I face this issue with my patients on a regular basis. Unfortunately, for young women and men facing a diagnosis of cancer, the issue of future fertility is often not addressed or even considered when discussing treatment options. The overwhelming anxiety of the cancer diagnosis eclipses other considerations for patients, and physicians have focused on the immediacy of cancer therapy rather than the ability to have children later in life. For some patients, the concern about losing fertility may adversely impact decisions about treatment, potentially leading young adults to choose less-than-ideal therapies. In this book, Gina Shaw presents a detailed and thoughtful guide to a variety of approaches for preserving future fertility for both women and men, as well as a detailed list of options for becoming parents when having a biological child is not possible.

Although current chemotherapy regimens for many cancers cause relatively less permanent damage to the function of the ovaries or testicles than treatments given in the past, the impact of chemotherapy, hormone therapies, and radiation on the subsequent ability to have children is largely unknown and is extremely complex. Some treatments are known to cause permanent loss of ovarian function or sperm production in all patients (such as whole body radiation), but most affect a subset of individuals. Risk factors include the type and duration of chemotherapy, patient age (particularly for women), and fertility before treatment, which is often unknown. Although there is information about risk factors that predict persistent loss of menses after chemotherapy and radiation, there is little data on the impact of these treatments as well as antihormone therapy on what is referred to in women as "ovarian reserve," making it difficult or impossible to accurately predict the effect of many anticancer therapies on fertility for an individual patient. For women, many therapies lead to a temporary cessation of menses. Whether menses restart, and whether fertility will remain intact, remains a question for most patients. Very young women, or women and men receiving less intensive therapy, may retain fertility. Choices regarding treatment, and discussion of the potential impact of the chosen treatment on fertility, must take place as early as possible after diagnosis in order to maximize fertility preserving options.

Fertility is an established subspecialty within obstetrics and gynecology, but the interest in preserving options for childbearing in young patients with a diagnosis of potentially curable cancer has given rise to a specialty within fertility, termed "oncofertility" by many. This term encompasses both service in the form of rapidly attainable consultations, egg harvesting, in vitro fertilization, and other fertility treatments, as well as research into the effects of treatment on ovarian reserve and subsequent fertility. Newer tests can more accurately predict the "ovarian reserve" or the ovary's potential to make fertilizable eggs, and help to predict the chances of achieving an unassisted pregnancy. At the University of California, San Francisco, we work very closely with our colleagues specializing in fertility, obtaining consultations before patients start systemic therapy including chemotherapy and hormone therapy, as well as radiation, in order to maximize fertility options as much as is feasible for each interested patient. Once a consultation is obtained, the patient and her partner or family can decide on the most appropriate plan for that woman's individual situation. Harvesting eggs that are then fertilized with sperm and frozen as embryos (the process followed for in vitro fertilization, or IVF) is the most successful strategy but requires a partner or donor sperm. Many women who do not have a male partner are wary of using donor sperm but can now consider freezing unfertilized eggs, a process which is slowly becoming more common but is still associated with a lower success rate than IVF—although this is improving. As timing is critical in order to minimize the delay until the start of cancer therapy, and harvesting eggs is timed to the menstrual cycle, patients can usually be seen within one to two days of an initial call. As much as possible, we try to delay the start of chemotherapy and radiation therapy for these discussions and procedures to minimize effects on the ovaries. In most cases, a several week delay is both safe and feasible. Harvesting eggs is not for everyone, and options are discussed in this book for those who do not have this resource.

So, you have survived your cancer, and have recovered from the side effects of therapy. As a cancer survivor, is it safe or possible to have children? Safety issues are complex, and depend on the type of cancer, as well as whether or not hormones like estrogen can be potential growth factors for the cancer. However, misconceptions rather than factual information drive many of the recommendations given to prospective parents. *Having Children After Cancer* cannot provide individual risk information, but it does provide direction on the types of questions to ask your providers, and briefly reviews existing data as well as the opinions of a variety of experts in this area.

For a number of reasons, a diagnosis of breast cancer can make decisions regarding childbearing particularly difficult. First, many breast cancers respond to estrogen, and treatment to prevent recurrence includes estrogen-blocking agents given for at least five years following diagnosis. For women who are thirty-five or older at the start of therapy, this important treatment creates a dilemma in terms of maintenance of fertility, and attempting pregnancy. It is important to make a careful assessment of risk for cancer recurrence if treatment is curtailed, and weigh this against the risk of not being able to have children at an older age. For very low-risk cancers, the risk of recurrence may not be sufficient to delay an attempt at pregnancy, but the reverse is likely for higher risk disease. The author was not faced with this issue, due to the type of cancer she had, but details her decisions and concerns with her older age and exposure to chemotherapy. In addition, she discusses fertility issues for men, and those who received chemotherapy as children and are now adults.

Regardless of your situation, you should be able to discuss risks and benefits as well as ask appropriate questions of your oncologist. As Ms. Shaw outlines, existing data does not support a worse cancer outcome for women who have children after a cancer diagnosis, and for breast cancer patients, pregnancy may even be protective. However, for those who do not have this option, embryo or egg donation, surrogacy, and adoption are discussed with vignettes from real-life cancer survivors, some of whom are followed through several different experiences with both successes and failures. Ms. Shaw provides a number of resources, as well as an outline of different possibilities for adoption with a realistic assessment of each approach, and a detailed description of international adoptions by country.

Rarely, cancer is diagnosed during pregnancy, posing a special challenge to effective treatment. The good news is that certain chemotherapy agents appear to be safe after the first trimester. To document this, a recent series of patients with breast cancer diagnosed during pregnancy was presented at a national meeting and demonstrated healthy babies at the time of delivery. Longer term follow-up is more limited, but suggests no long-term impact to children exposed to a limited course of safe agents in utero. By giving chemotherapy before surgery, the cancer can be treated effectively without significant risk while the mother is still pregnant, allowing the baby to mature to term or near term. Treatment of cancer during pregnancy requires a specialist in the treatment of the specific cancer, as well as a high-risk obstetrician. For some patients with breast cancer, delaying surgery and proceeding with chemotherapy can allow for breast conservation following delivery.

In addition to discussing ways to preserve fertility, and options if pregnancy is not possible, *Having Children After Cancer* includes a chapter on how to stay healthy if you are a pregnant cancer survivor. The author discusses many challenges including poor or absent milk production from a breast which has received radiation to treat cancer, cancer screening, what to do and issues to consider if you get pregnant while taking antihormone therapy for cancer, as well as other topics. As in the other chapters, most situations are illustrated by real people's experiences and decisions, as well as the opinions of experts. These "pearls" of information are an invaluable resource to a woman facing these issues, and most oncologists are not particularly knowledgeable about these topics.

Many of our patients are also parents, often of younger children. And if you do have children after a cancer diagnosis, you are still a cancer survivor—having faced your own mortality is a sobering reminder of the short and unpredictable nature of life. I love the chapter in this book titled, "What's Cancer, Mom?" Seventeen years ago I was a daughter, with a mother who had cancer. Although I was an adult with small children myself, and a young doctor, I wish both of us had had the advice in this section. Ms. Shaw quotes a child psychologist: "Make memories and make them concrete," and then goes on to provide her own suggestions about how to make this happen. I was pleased to see how these recommendations mirror those I give to my patients, and have taken to heart in my own family. The book ends with an important and heartfelt sentiment—building a family is "worth it all."

Two messages are critical. First, if you have been diagnosed with early-stage cancer and are facing treatment that could impact your fertility, except in very rare cases you have time to consider your options, talk with a fertility expert, and determine the best approach for you and, if existing, your partner. Although the cost of many options can seem more than daunting, be empowered to explore funding sources. This book provides direction, resources, and even advice on how to approach insurance companies (who generally do not cover fertility treatment). Second, there are many routes to pursue in the road to becoming a parent, so if possible, keep your options and mind open.

A cancer diagnosis does not *have* to close the door to future fertility or the experience of parenting. This book provides an invaluable guide to a subject previously relegated to the backstage in the field of oncology. As more patients are cured of early-stage cancer, issues critical to quality of life for survivors, such as fertility, have moved closer to center stage. Read this book, learn more, use available resources, and ask questions!

—*Hope S. Rugo, MD, medical oncologist specializing in breast cancer and professor of medicine, University of California, San Francisco, Helen Diller Family Comprehensive Cancer Center*

Having Children After Cancer

The Joy and the Worry

WHEN I ANNOUNCED TO friends and family that I was pregnant for the first time at age forty, the responses were predictably jubilant. My father nearly dropped the phone, then yelled "Oh no! Oh YES! *Dorothy!*" as he bellowed for my mom to join the conversation. When we surprised my in-laws with an unexpected visit and an ultrasound picture, my mother-in-law burst into happy tears.

But as a breast cancer survivor, I wasn't surprised when I got some other, more cautious responses as well. A couple of people ventured to ask if this was definitely a good thing. My friend Lisa, after rejoicing with me in an email headed "OMG OMG OMG OMG!" tentatively asked, "Without intending to be a buzzkill—does this increase the risk of the cancer returning?"

When you're diagnosed with breast cancer two weeks before your thirty-seventh birthday, all kinds of things are different—and pregnancy is one of them.

When I was first diagnosed in 2004, the doctors offered the option of freezing eggs prior to starting chemotherapy, in case I wanted to try and get pregnant afterward. I said no. I had gone through enough medical procedures already and was about to start even more, and the last thing I wanted was more poking and prodding. I also didn't want to delay the inevitable chemotherapy longer than I had to. Let's just get started, please.

Plus, I was scared of getting pregnant after cancer. For most people who've had cancer during their reproductive years, the big issue is, *can* you get pregnant (or get someone else pregnant) after chemotherapy or radiation have beaten up your system? But for women who've had breast cancer, the added (and perhaps even bigger) question is, *should* you? In 2006, my husband and I adopted our daughter in domestic open adoption, in part because we thought I probably couldn't get pregnant after cancer and in part because we feared that maybe I shouldn't.

That's because breast cancer often feeds on hormones, and there's nothing like pregnancy for sending your body's hormone production into overdrive. If you think you've treated your breast cancer successfully, there still may be tiny *micrometastases*—areas where cancer has spread, but is still too small to see—lurking somewhere in your body, indolent and nonthreatening for the moment. Could pregnancy wake them up?

The answer to that question, and to my friend Lisa's similar one, is "Nobody really knows for sure." To date, most studies have shown that there's no increased risk of cancer recurrence for women who get pregnant; in fact, a literature review published in the *European Journal of Cancer* in 2003 found that overall survival in women who got pregnant after breast cancer compared favorably with those who didn't.[1] That, however, may be explained by the "healthy subject" bias—if you're healthy enough to try and get pregnant after breast cancer, that probably means you aren't one of the women who had a very early recurrence of your disease (within the first year or so). And those are all small studies. Because breast cancer in women under forty-five is relatively rare (about 24,000 women in that age group are diagnosed every year, compared with about 180,000 women over forty-five) and pregnancy after breast cancer is even rarer, that means it's hard to recruit many women for research.

My breast surgeon, Jeanne Petrek, was one of the nation's leading experts in breast cancer in younger women, and she headed up the largest prospective study to examine this question. Her study looked at both issues—premature menopause in young women with breast cancer (how likely is it that the menopause will be permanent?) and pregnancy in those same women (how risky is it?).

Dr. Petrek told me that although the small studies showed no risk, biologically speaking, there *should* be an increased risk. That didn't mean she was telling me or any other breast cancer survivor not to get pregnant—just that we needed to know there were still unanswered questions, which she hoped her study would help to answer.

Her study is still ongoing, led by another doctor because Dr. Petrek died in a tragic car accident in Manhattan in 2005. The menopause results came out a year or so later, but it will take longer to really know if the women enrolled in the study who got pregnant after cancer then developed recurrences at a higher rate than those who didn't get pregnant.

Studies aside, my biological clock wasn't just ticking, it was chiming the hour. Waiting another year or two or five for the results was, I figured, effectively deciding not to get pregnant. So in the spring of 2007, my husband and I decided to throw caution to the wind. We wanted another child desperately and were thinking of starting the adoption process again. But before we did, we decided to try getting pregnant—since no doctor, no test, had ever told us it definitely wouldn't be possible. How did I get to that point, after being so terrified of the prospect prior to treatment that I hadn't bothered to freeze eggs in case "chemopause" became permanent?

First, I had experienced a remarkable response to treatment—something called a *complete pathological response*, which meant that when the doctors went in to remove what was left of my breast lump after initial chemotherapy, it was gone. Nothing but benign tissue remained. Every time I mention this to any breast specialist, they ooh and aah over how lucky that was. It's considered the best predictor of whether or not your cancer will come back.

Second, it had been three years since treatment, and my watchful doctors had spotted no sign of recurrence. Those were the riskiest years for women with my form of breast cancer, and I'd made it through them safely. I had also had "hormone-negative" disease, meaning my cancer wasn't fed by estrogen or progesterone, and so I hadn't been prescribed a five-year course of the drug Tamoxifen. That would have required a tough decision about whether to go off the drug to become pregnant—a dilemma many women face, which I'll discuss later in the book. I did spend a year taking the drug Herceptin, because my tumor was positive for a protein called Her2/neu, but I was done with that by the time we started talking about pregnancy.

Third—well, there's no real third, not exactly. The first two factors were real, specific items about my risk that I could weigh and consider. The third factor was totally intangible: my desire to experience pregnancy and childbirth. I love my daughter with all my heart and soul, and I wish more than anything that I could have carried her inside me and given birth to her—but of course, that would have made her a different child from the perfect one she is.

While she was pregnant, our daughter's birth mother told me that she so hoped that I could get pregnant someday so that I could experience this. I told her it would be all right if I didn't—and it would have been. And if there had been some piece of paper telling me that I would definitely double my risk of the cancer coming back if I did get pregnant, maybe I wouldn't have. But the answer to that question was unknown, and putting an unknown fear against a deep and real desire to have a baby, I chose not to worry (too much) about the unknown.

Once I got through my constant first-trimester fears of miscarriage, my pregnancy was a joyous and largely easy experience. My oncologist was so unworried about the risks that when I asked if she needed me to come in for a visit sooner than my usual appointment, she said, "Nah. See you in December." On March 11, 2008, my son, Adrian, was born—a healthy, cuddly little boy whom we never could have imagined existing just three years earlier. And unbelievably enough, less than two years later—at what some might consider the reproductively decrepit age of forty-two—we conceived again. In June 2010, our daughter Katia joined her big brother and sister to make us a family of five.

Some people might say I made a foolish decision, took a crazy risk when we could have adopted again, risked leaving my daughter without a mother at a young age. I think that I decided to choose faith: faith in my body, faith in my instincts, faith in my future. And anyone who's ever had cancer knows that those things can often seem to be lost when you face this disease. Having my son and new daughter means I've got my faith in life back, and bringing them into this world is my promise to them and their big sister that I intend to be here for a long, long time.

Every year, thousands of men and women who are diagnosed with—and overcome—cancer in their reproductive years face many of the same questions and fears I faced—and many more of their own—while at the same time nurturing hopes for a child, or more children. We take different paths. Some pursue one of the many and growing avenues for assisted reproduction. Others choose adoption—domestic, international, or through foster care. Others hope for natural conception. Whatever path we take to become parents, it's a much harder one than that traveled by the lucky folks who've never heard the three words no one wants to hear: "You have cancer."

My experience was with breast cancer, but treatment for any kind of cancer can put your fertility at risk. All of the active treatments for testicular cancer—which strikes more than eight thousand men in the United States each year, most of them under forty-five—are known to damage fertility. Treatments for endometrial cancer and ovarian cancer usually involve removal of the uterus or ovaries—effectively putting a halt to a woman's childbearing years.

But your cancer doesn't have to be related to your reproductive system to put your hopes of having a child in jeopardy. Chemotherapy and radiation for leukemia, Hodgkin's disease, melanoma, and many other types of cancer can damage sperm and eggs. And when a young child is diagnosed with cancer, their parents must add worries about their son's or daughter's ability to have their own children someday to an already endless list of fears.

Cancer survivors who want a family wonder about so many things. Should we delay cancer treatment a few weeks so that we can preserve eggs? Is it safe to choose a newer, "fertility-sparing" method of treatment? How do we tell a home study agency, or an expectant mother considering us as adoptive parents for her baby, that one of us had cancer? How much of a risk is it to get pregnant after having breast cancer? What if the cancer returns while I'm pregnant? Am I putting my children at risk of losing their mother or father early?

There are no simple answers to these questions. But this book is designed to walk you through all of your options for having children after cancer—and there are many! We'll talk about everything from how to preserve your fertility while undergoing treatment to what countries are friendliest to cancer survivors seeking to adopt internationally (an often-changing list) to what your financial options are and when, if, and how to talk to your children about having had cancer.

This book gives you both scientific and professional information from top experts in the field, as well as been-there–done-that insights from women and men who have faced these decisions themselves.

Cancer steals so much from so many of us: our health, our peace of mind, our confidence in our bodies, and of course at its worst, months and years of our lives. It shouldn't be able to steal our hopes for a family as well. If you want to have a child, or more children, there's no reason that a cancer diagnosis should close the door to those dreams.

CHAPTER 1

Cancer and the Chance of Children

How Cancer Treatments Affect Your Fertility

CANCER IS THE THIEF that keeps on taking. At its very worst, of course, it can take your life. But even if it doesn't, it can take a lot of other things—everything from your hair and your ability to enjoy a pizza to your energy, your sex drive, your memory, and your sense of confidence in yourself and your body. Some of those things you get back after cancer treatment, and some may never return entirely. (I've heard some people call cancer a gift, but if my cancer was a gift, I'd like to know where the return desk is.)

Just when you think you know all of the things cancer can steal from you, there's another: your fertility. About half of all people diagnosed with cancer in their reproductive years receive treatments that can impair fertility: chemotherapy that can attack your supply of remaining eggs, radiation that zaps sperm inside the testicles, and hormonal treatments that shut down your menstrual cycle and throw you into premature menopause.

But when the doctor says, "It's cancer" (don't we all remember the exact moment when we first heard those words that yanked the rug right out from under us?), you're not thinking, "What will this do to my ability to have children?" You're thinking, "Oh my God, am I going to die?"

Then you're thinking about more tests and biopsies and surgeries and chemotherapy appointments and whether you're going to need a wig or not and are you going to be throwing up all the time and how are you going to tell parents, kids, bosses, and coworkers? You're fretting about health insurance coverage. You're worrying about whether the disease has spread to the lymph nodes or metastasized to other organs. You're wondering if you'll ever, ever go a minute or an hour—much less a day or a week—without the constant refrain of "IhavecancerIhavecancerIhavecancer" drumming away inside your head.

If you're a parent with a young child who's just been diagnosed with cancer, you're enduring all of these worries for your child and at the same time wondering how you're going to be strong for her when you can barely make it through the day without breaking down.

So at a time like this, it's little wonder that a lot of people don't stop to think about, or ask about, what cancer might mean for their ability to have children in the future—even though it's something they may care deeply about. And most cancer specialists, who have to impart a lot of information about their patients' illness and treatment options in a very short time, don't focus on fertility either.

In fact, a national survey of oncologists conducted in 2008 found that although about two-thirds discuss the issue of fertility with newly diagnosed patients, less than 25 percent referred their patients to a fertility specialist or provided educational materials about what risks cancer treatment might pose to fertility and what options patients might have.[1]

> **ASK YOUR DOCTOR**
>
> Teresa Woodruff, who heads the national Oncofertility Consortium headquartered at Northwestern University, recommends that you ask your doctor—or your child's—these five questions:[2]
>
> 1. How is my cancer affecting my health right now?
> 2. How quickly do I need to start treatment?
> 3. Will my cancer or its treatment affect my future fertility?
> 4. What fertility options are out there?
> 5. Can I have a child after my cancer?

The problem is, you don't have a lot of time to educate yourself about what might happen to your fertility—or your child's—as a result of cancer treatment. You're making decisions about treatment with visions of a window that's rapidly closing, fearing that every day you delay allows the cancer to spread. So you need information, and you need it fast. That's what this book is for. Keep reading.

What Cancer Does to Your Fertility

Just how does cancer affect your fertility? Sometimes, it's the cancer itself that does the damage. For example, researchers have found that two of every three male patients with Hodgkin's lymphoma have impaired sperm production before they even start treatment, although no one yet knows exactly why this is.[3] Testicular cancer can also disrupt normal hormonal levels in men, leading to limited or abnormal sperm production; and at least one recent study has suggested that men with fertility problems may be at increased risk for developing testicular cancer in the first place.[4] Experts have speculated that this could be because their mothers' exposures to certain hormones during pregnancy triggered cell malformations that later showed up in the adult men as fertility problems and testicular cancer.

Women who carry the breast cancer 1 (BRCA1) mutation—the most common genetic mutation associated with breast cancer—may have impaired fertility even if they haven't yet been diagnosed with an actual cancer. Recent research indicates that women with BRCA1 could have lower ovarian reserve (fewer eggs) than other women. Kutluk Oktay, MD, a pioneer in the field of cancer and fertility, has found that the ovarian reserve in his patients with breast cancer, but without a BRCA1 mutation, can be as much as thirty-eight times higher than the egg reserve in women with BRCA1.[5] "The women in our study who had low response to ovarian stimulation were all thirty-three and older, so this is probably an effect that catches up in your thirties," Oktay says. "For those who attempt pregnancy early on, it may not be a big issue, but if you delay childbearing, then it may catch up." He advises women who want children and know they have a BRCA1 mutation to consult with a fertility specialist, even if they have not yet been diagnosed with cancer themselves.

Usually, though, it's the treatment that attacks your fertility, not the cancer itself and not a gene associated with it. Doctors tend to pursue the most aggressive treatments possible in younger cancer patients—because they have a lot more years of life to preserve, because younger and healthier patients are strong enough to withstand more intense side effects, and because cancer in young people is often more aggressive than cancer in older people. It makes perfect sense. But it also means that these toxic treatments have a particularly high chance of impairing fertility.

As you're making treatment decisions, it's important to know how individual drugs and treatment regimens can affect your ability to have children. You're not going to refuse lifesaving chemotherapy or surgery just because they might damage your fertility—or you shouldn't—but you *may* be able to choose modifications to your treatment regimen. And in the next chapter, we'll talk about a growing list of fertility-preserving technologies available to both men and women, before and during treatment. Your decisions about whether to pursue some of these options might also be affected by just how toxic your particular treatments are likely to be.

Chemotherapy

Chemotherapy drugs are stupid drugs. That is, they attack blindly and indiscriminately, killing healthy and diseased cells alike. Their target: anything that's dividing too rapidly. Cancer cells divide more rapidly than most other cells, but so do hair follicle cells and the cells that line your gastrointestinal tract—hence the baldies and the barfies that accompany many chemotherapy regimens.

The cells that nurse a woman's eggs to maturity—the somatic cells—are also dividing more rapidly than other cells, while the immature eggs themselves are also particularly vulnerable to DNA damage. So chemotherapy can often put women into premature menopause. This chemopause is sometimes temporary and sometimes permanent. In general, the younger you are when you receive chemotherapy, the more likely you are to either maintain a normal menstrual cycle during treatment or get your periods back once chemo is over. That's because the younger you are, the more eggs you have left. Women are born with all the eggs we'll ever have—about a million at birth and about one hundred thousand by the time we reach puberty.

Sperm production is also very sensitive to chemotherapy. Men make millions of sperm every day, so it's not like sperm are a finite resource (as with a woman's eggs). But sperm are constantly developing, maturing, and reproducing, making them a prime target for those "stupid" chemotherapy drugs.

Not all chemotherapy drugs are created equal when it comes to fertility. The class of drugs that wreaks the most havoc on your ability to conceive children—whether you're a man or a woman—is known as *alkylating agents*. The most commonly used of these drugs is called Cytoxan (cyclophosphamide). If you're under forty-five and have had chemotherapy for breast cancer, you've almost certainly been given Cytoxan; it's also used to treat lymphoma and some forms of leukemia. It can do irreversible damage to both immature eggs and sperm. The longer you take Cytoxan, or any of its sibling drugs, the more likely you are to have permanent damage to your fertility.

Other chemotherapy drugs can impair your fertility as well, but they're much less toxic—to your gonads, at least. Adriamycin (doxorubicin), another very common breast cancer drug, is considered to be an intermediate, or moderate, fertility risk in women over forty and only a minimal risk for younger women. Methotrexate and 5-FU, often used to treat a host of cancers, are thought to pose very little threat to fertility—at least by themselves. These drugs are often delivered as part of a "chemo cocktail" with other medications that can have a greater fertility risk.

And then, of course, there's a long list of drugs we just don't know much about in terms of what they do to your ability to bear children. The taxanes—known as Taxol (paclitaxel) and Taxotere (docetaxel)—don't appear to damage fertility at all, but doctors still don't know for sure. The same can be said of oxaliplatin and irinotecan, used to treat ovarian cancer and colon cancer. See the chart starting on page 15, "Chemotherapy Drugs and Fertility," for more information.

But even if you get the most toxic of chemotherapy drugs, that doesn't mean your ability to conceive a child will vanish forever. Your hair almost always comes back, even after the most toxic chemo (although it often looks different); sometimes, your reproductive abilities can too.

For women, most of the time it's a numbers game—that is, it's all about age (frustrating, but true). When I was treated for breast cancer in 2004, at thirty-six, my doctor, an expert on young women with cancer, told me that I had about a fifty-fifty chance of coming out of chemopause within a few months of treatment ending. Had I been in my early thirties or younger, she said, she'd have given me even better odds. The closer a woman gets to forty, or even older, the lower her chances are of getting her period back or conceiving a child, she said.

But since then, some studies have come out that are more encouraging. An Israeli study released at the 2009 meeting of the American Society of Clinical Oncology found that almost all of a group of sixty-five breast cancer patients thirty-eight and younger got their periods back after treatment, and about a third of them—nearly 34 percent—became pregnant.[6]

The picture is cloudier, though, for women undergoing chemo over age forty—studies indicate that the chances of getting your menstrual cycle back at this age are anywhere from 5 to 20 percent.[7] In general, if you're a woman diagnosed with cancer at or after age forty and still want to have children after treatment, the odds are pretty strong that you won't be able to conceive spontaneously—you'll likely either have to use assisted reproduction methods, adoption, or surrogacy.

But if you're under forty at diagnosis and treatment, your chances of getting pregnant later on may be better than you think. Michelle Rommelfanger, already the mother of twin boys, was twenty-nine when she was diagnosed with stage II breast cancer. She underwent the classic breast cancer treatment for young women like her: four rounds of Adriamycin (doxorubicin) and Cytoxan and four rounds of Taxol, followed by radiation and the hormonal drug Tamoxifen. While on Tamoxifen, she discovered that her IUD had failed and she was pregnant. She later delivered a healthy baby girl, Mira (short for miracle) Eliana.

"It was a very scary and hard road for a couple of weeks, but she is a miracle baby!" she says. "I was excited and scared all in one, but I refuse to live in fear of the beast. This happened for a reason—this baby was determined to be here!" (There'll be more on Michelle later in the book.)

For men, age is not as much of an issue. Since new sperm are constantly being "born," it's not like chemotherapy can kill off all of a guy's remaining swimmers. "The number of sperm produced with every heartbeat is like ten to the fifth power, so even if you damage half of that, it's not a huge impact," says Dr. Woodruff. "There certainly are treatments that can be completely sterilizing for a man, no matter what his age, but men are generally less vulnerable to chemotherapy than women when it comes to fertility."

Whether you're a man or a woman, twenty-eight or thirty-eight, can you ask *not* to be given a specific drug that's known to be particularly bad for fertility? For example, the "gold standard" chemotherapy regimen for breast cancer is known as AC-T: a combination of Adriamycin (doxorubicin) and Cytoxan, followed by a taxane (Taxol or Taxotere). The only drug in this cocktail that's known to do significant damage to your chances of bearing children is Cytoxan—so can you ask your doctor just to drop the C and give you the A-T instead?

You can ask, but your doctor will most likely say no—at least for right now. Some doctors *have* proposed a breast cancer regimen without the Cytoxan, to preserve fertility—it was brought up at the San Antonio Breast Cancer Symposium in 2007, for example—but for now, AC-T remains the gold standard for most younger women with invasive breast cancers. "Today, they're still going to use it," says Dr. Woodruff. Similarly, other cancers may have multiple chemo modalities, but there may be a very good reason that your oncologist insists you must receive the one that is more toxic to your fertility. "But ultimately," reassures Dr. Woodruff, "yes, we want to come up with smarter chemotherapies that can treat the disease and leave the rest of the body alone."

Some doctors have suggested ovarian suppression and other chemical means of protecting fertility during chemotherapy, but the science just isn't there yet (see chapter 2, page 49). In the meantime, there are fertility-preserving measures you can take before undergoing chemotherapy, which we will discuss in the next chapter.

CHEMOTHERAPY DRUGS AND FERTILITY

What are some of the most common chemotherapy drugs and treatment regimens, and what might they do to your fertility? Find out here.[8] (The chart also includes a few medications that are not technically chemotherapy but are instead monoclonal antibodies and other targeted therapies.)

Drug: ABVD (a combination of Adriamycin, bleomycin, vinblastine, and dacarbazine)
Used for: First-line treatment of Hodgkin's lymphoma
Risk: Minimal for both men and women. Less than 20 percent of women develop permanent amenorrhea after treatment, and men usually have a temporary loss of sperm production.

Drug: AC (Adriamycin and cyclophosphamide)
Used for: Breast cancer
Risk: Low risk for women under forty, with less than a 20 percent chance of permanent infertility. For women over forty, estimates vary; you may have between a 30 and 70 percent chance of losing fertility permanently after AC. (AC is not generally used in cancers affecting men.) But keep in mind that most of the time, AC is

delivered in combination with P or T—Paclitaxel or Taxotere, taxane drugs that can have an additional impact on fertility. When the regimen is AC-T or AC-P, risk of loss of fertility rises to between 29 and 42 percent for women under forty, and 66 to 77 percent for women over forty.

Drug: BEAM (BCNU, etoposide, cytosine arabinoside, melphalan) and any other chemotherapy regimen used to prepare for bone marrow transplantation
Used for: Preparation for bone marrow transplantation, in cancers such as leukemias, lymphomas, and some solid tumors
Risk: High for both men and women. Most chemotherapy regimens associated with bone marrow transplants present a major risk of permanent infertility.

Drug: Bevacizumab (Avastin)
Used for: Colon cancer and non-small-cell lung cancer
Risk: There is still limited research information on precisely how bevacizumab may affect fertility, but in animal studies, bevacizumab disrupts menstrual cycles and interferes with follicular development, a side effect that at least sometimes persists after treatment. The drug's manufacturer lists impaired fertility as a known side effect. How significant the risk of permanent infertility or sterility is remains unknown.

Drug: CAF (cyclophosphamide, doxorubicin, 5-FU), CEF (cyclophosphamide, epirubicin, 5-FU), or CMF (cyclophosphamide, methotrexate, 5-fluorouracil)
Used for: Breast cancer

Risk: Low risk of permanent loss of fertility in women under thirty (less than 20 percent). Intermediate risk in women in their thirties (30 to 70 percent). For women over forty, this combination is high risk, causing amenorrhea in more than 80 percent of patients.

Drug: Cetuximab (Erbitux)
Used for: Colon cancer, head and neck cancer
Risk: Very little is known about cetuximab's impact on fertility in humans. Some animal studies have shown interference with menstrual cycles, including an absence of cycles altogether, but it's not known how long that lasts after treatment is discontinued.

Drug: CHOP (cyclophosphamide, doxorubicin, vincristine, prednisone)
Used for: Non-Hodgkin's lymphoma
Risk: Low risk.

Drug: COPP (cyclophosphamide, vincristine, procarbazine, prednisone) and COPP/ABVD
Used for: Hodgkin's lymphoma
Risk: Both regimens pose a very high risk to fertility, leaving 80 percent of women with permanent amenorrhea and men with prolonged loss of sperm production.

Drug: Cyclophosphamide alone, at higher doses, or for bone marrow transplant conditioning
Used for: Sarcoma, non-Hodgkin's lymphoma, acute lymphocytic leukemia (ALL), and neuroblastoma
Risk: There is a high risk of permanent infertility or sterility for both men and women.

Drug: Docetaxel (Taxol, Taxotere)
Used for: Breast cancer
Risk: Not completely researched, but so far all the taxane drugs seem to pose relatively low risk to fertility.

Drug: Erlotinib (Tarceva)
Used for: Non-small-cell lung cancer, pancreatic cancer
Risk: Little is known about Tarceva's risk to fertility in either men and women. In animal studies, the drug did not impair fertility in either male or female rats.

Drug: Imatinib (Gleevec)
Used for: Chronic myeloid leukemia (CML), gastrointestinal stromal tumor (GIST)
Risk: There has not been a lot of research on fertility after Gleevec, but a number of women have become pregnant after being treated with this drug. Interestingly, Gleevec may also have potential in fertility *preservation* during cancer treatment—see chapter 2 for more on this.

Drug: MOPP (nitrogen mustard, vincristine, procarabazine, prednisone) or MVPP (nitrogen mustard, vinblastine, prednisone, procarbazine)
Used for: Hodgkin's lymphoma
Risk: High risk of permanent loss of fertility.

Drug: NOVP (mitoxantrone, vincristine, vinblastine, prednisone)
Used for: Hodgkin's lymphoma
Risk: There is a low risk of permanent loss of fertility.

Drug: Oxaliplatin (Eloxatin)
Used for: Ovarian cancer, colon cancer
Risk: There has not been a lot of research on the fertility effects of oxaliplatin, but preclinical studies in animals did show some negative impact on menstrual cycles and testicular function, which could persist after treatment.

Drug: Procarbazine
Used for: Hodgkin's lymphoma
Risk: There is a high risk of permanent infertility.

Drug: Trastuzumab (Herceptin)
Used for: Breast cancer
Risk: Not a lot of research has been done on Herceptin and fertility, but experts note that it is a very selective drug and there is no evidence that it damages eggs.

Radiation

Radiation is a much more targeted treatment than chemotherapy. Radiation oncologists design your radiation field so that it will hit the cancer cells as precisely as possible and spare the surrounding tissues and organs. But when the cancer is within your reproductive organs, or very nearby, it's hard to keep the radiation from damaging them.

Types of cancer that can require radiation to the pelvic area include

- Cervical cancer

- Ovarian cancer

- Endometrial cancer

- Testicular cancer

- Prostate cancer

- Colorectal cancer

Irradiating a woman's gynecologic organs can impair fertility in a couple of different ways. First, it can actually injure the ovaries and prevent them from releasing healthy, mature eggs for fertilization. Radiation can also scar the uterus, making it harder to sustain a pregnancy once it's conceived and putting you at increased risk of miscarriage and other complications. Just as with chemotherapy, the higher the dose of radiation you get, and the longer you get it, the likelier you are to have impaired fertility.

"The location of the tumor makes a big difference in whether fertility is damaged by radiation," explains Karine Chung, MD, the founder and director of the fertility preservation program at the University of Southern California. "For example, if you're having radiation to the breast or the spine at neck level, we can protect you from radiation scatter with shielding. But if the tumor is in the abdomen, right next to the ovaries, it's very difficult to shield them."[9]

A man's testicles are particularly vulnerable to radiation damage. Even very low doses can impact sperm production and formation, and the longer the dose of radiation, the greater and longer-lasting the damage is. Extremely high doses of radiation to the pelvic area can leave a man totally sterile.

Radiation dosage is measured in *grays* (Gy). In men, direct radiation to the testicles of more than 2.5 Gy cumulatively poses a high risk for permanent sterility; but if the radiation is directed at another part of the body—say, the abdomen—and the testicles only get scattered radiation, doses as high as 5 or 6 Gy may not leave a man permanently sterile. In adult women, abdominal or pelvic radiation doses of 6 Gy or greater pose a high risk for permanent infertility.

Some cancers, like leukemias, may also be treated with total body irradiation (TBI), which can be devastating to the ability to father or bear children. Research has found that the younger a man is when he receives TBI, the more likely it is that he may recover some ability to generate healthy sperm.[10]

Sometimes radiation can affect fertility even if it's not aimed at your pelvis. If you're receiving radiotherapy for a brain tumor or another type of head and neck cancer, for example, the radiation could affect the functioning of your pituitary gland, which helps to control your ovarian cycle.

In the event that radiation must be directed toward the pelvis, there is an option for surgically moving the ovaries out of the line of fire. This procedure, called *ovarian transposition*, is discussed in the next chapter (see page 51).

Surgery

There are a number of cancers that involve the reproductive organs—cervical, ovarian, and endometrial cancer for women and prostate and testicular cancer for men. Surgery for any of these cancers can mean taking out something that's vital to getting pregnant or getting someone else pregnant. Uterine cancer, for example, almost always requires a complete hysterectomy. Women with ovarian cancer and men with testicular cancer, depending on the stage of the disease, might lose only one ovary or testicle to surgery, or both might have to be removed. For information on possible fertility-sparing surgical options—including removing only one ovary or testicle, avoiding a radical hysterectomy, or waiting to remove the uterus until after a pregnancy—see chapter 2, pages 34, 51, and 53.

Thinking way ahead, surgery for breast cancer can also damage the breast's ability to lactate. If you are planning a lumpectomy and want to preserve the prospect of nursing a child later, ask your surgeon if he or she can make a surgical plan that will spare the milk ducts as much as possible. Most, if not all, young women who have breast-conserving surgery also have radiation, which damages the breast's ability to lactate. (You'll learn more about this in chapter 6.) So it may be unlikely that you'll be able to breast-feed on that side anyway. If this is very important to you, however, it's worth at least asking your doctor about your options. And remember, some women have very successfully nursed with only one fully lactating breast!

Hormonal Treatments

If you've been diagnosed with the kind of breast cancer that is stimulated by the levels of female hormones in the body—specifically, estrogen and progesterone—you'll probably be prescribed hormonal therapies for at least a year, and up to five years, after your initial treatment, to reduce your risk of recurrence. Premenopausal women usually take a drug called Tamoxifen, although there are other drugs that are options after menopause.

It's not yet know whether or not Tamoxifen damages fertility. It might reduce ovarian reserves over time, and studies are now being done to try to answer this question. In at least some cases, though, it does the opposite. At higher doses, Tamoxifen is sometimes used as a fertility treatment, because it often *increases* ovulation. About 20 percent of women taking Tamoxifen will experience irregular periods while on the drug, but cycles usually go back to normal once Tamoxifen therapy stops, unless you were on the verge of menopause anyway.

The problem is that it is not considered safe to take Tamoxifen while pregnant. (Women who use this drug to amp up ovulation stop taking it once they conceive.) So that means that if you've been prescribed Tamoxifen, you have to wait until the end of your time on the drug to try to have a baby—and most doctors put women on Tamoxifen for five years. If you're already in your mid-thirties, waiting that long could close your window of fertility entirely.

Some women do put off hormonal treatments for cancer in order to get pregnant. That's what Jilda Nettleton did. She was diagnosed with breast cancer the day before her thirty-eighth birthday and underwent a lumpectomy and started radiation treatment the same month. But she had already been trying to get pregnant for over a year and decided to forego Tamoxifen until the next year, when her first daughter was born.

After a year on Tamoxifen, she went off the drug again and began to try to conceive her second child. A year later, her second daughter was born—and less than a year after that, she had a cancer recurrence and opted for a mastectomy. "Did I get a second cancer because of two pregnancies and only one year of Tamoxifen? Who knows?" she asks.

Most doctors strongly recommend taking Tamoxifen for at least two years after initial treatment before stopping the drug and trying to become pregnant, no matter how much you might want to try sooner. Research has shown that the overall duration of hormone therapy is important in helping to reduce late recurrences of breast cancer, so keep this in mind. Your doctor will also be able to give you more specific advice about what a "break" from Tamoxifen to get pregnant may mean for you as an individual, given factors such as your stage at diagnosis and the biology of your tumor. "Ideally, you should complete five years of Tamoxifen, but the reality is that a lot of women who want to get pregnant don't have that luxury of time," says M. Catherine Lee, MD, a breast specialist who focuses on fertility and breast cancer at Florida's H. Lee Moffitt Cancer Center. "There's no data to offer about 'taking a break' from Tamoxifen after two or three years and getting pregnant. We just don't know. For some women, that unknown is too much. Others say the clock is ticking. It's your body and your life, and you have to live it."[11]

Christina Demosthenous, diagnosed with stage I breast cancer at age thirty-two, did just that. After a lumpectomy, chemotherapy, radiation, and two years of Tamoxifen, she got pregnant on her first try. "I was never regular to begin with, and my cycles had stopped toward the end of chemo but returned two months later," she says. "I think some Tamoxifen in the beginning is better than none. The first few years after the diagnosis are critical."

In chapter 6, you'll read more about Michelle Rommelfanger, who became pregnant while taking Tamoxifen, and two other women who became pregnant while on other cancer therapies.

Monoclonal Antibodies

Here's where things get really murky. If you think there's not enough research out there on what standard treatments like chemotherapy do to your ability to have children, you haven't seen anything yet. *Monoclonal antibodies*—new, "smart" drugs that attack specific cancer-causing mutations like heat-seeking missiles—have revolutionized the treatment of some cancers, but we don't yet know for sure what they do to fertility, if anything.

It makes sense to think that these drugs—which include Herceptin for breast cancer, Avastin for colon and lung cancers, and Erbitux for colon and head and neck cancers—might not affect fertility at all. After all, they're not stupid drugs like chemotherapy. They're designed to hit their target and not damage other cells just because they happen to be growing fast. "These treatments are really specific," says Dr. Woodruff. "Our instinct is that cancer patients who take these drugs should be in a better position to retain their fertility."

Another newer drug, Gleevec, has had a dramatic impact on the lives of people with chronic myelogenous leukemia, many of them young. Gleevec is taken on a long-term basis—years at a stretch—and often induces a complete remission of the disease.

As compared to other treatments for leukemia, Gleevec appears to do little to no harm to the reproductive system. It also seems to be safe to conceive while taking the drug, but because it's not considered safe to take *while* pregnant, you'd have to go off Gleevec— and risk going out of remission (and potentially having trouble returning to remission once you start taking the drug again).

Since these drugs are all relatively new, less is known about all the side effects that may be identified once hundreds of thousands of patients have taken them over a number of years. Herceptin, for example, can do damage to heart function in a very small but still significant percentage of the women who take it. It's taken thousands of women and lots of clinical trials to discover that important fact, and it will take a *lot* longer and a lot more patients to know with certainty if any of these targeted therapies have any effect on fertility. In general, though, if you ask most cancer specialists today, they'll tell you that these drugs are not likely to do long-term damage to your ability to bear or father children.

Childhood Cancers

The picture for all of these treatments is a little different when it involves cancer in children, especially those who haven't yet reached puberty.

By far the most common childhood cancer is leukemia, which accounts for about one out of every three cancer cases in kids under the age of fifteen. Other common childhood cancers include central nervous system (CNS) malignancies, lymphomas, soft tissue sarcoma, renal cancer, and bone tumors. Almost all of these cancers are treated with alkylating chemotherapy, the most toxic to fertility in both men and women. For some young people with acute myelogenous leukemia (AML), a bone marrow transplant is lifesaving but can completely eradicate fertility.

Because they are much younger, girls do have a better chance than adult women of retaining their ability to bear children after cancer treatment—but they're still at risk. A large study of more than three thousand survivors of childhood cancer and their siblings found that girls who'd been treated for cancer were thirteen times more likely to go into premature menopause as adults than their sisters were.[12] Now, let's put that in perspective: it means 8 percent of cancer survivors went into premature menopause, which also means that 92 percent of them *didn't*. Just as with adults, the biggest risks are toxic chemotherapies (alkylating agents) and pelvic radiation—girls who had these treatments had a 30 percent chance of going through premature menopause.

The younger a girl is when she receives treatment, the more ovarian reserve she has—and the better chance she has of recovering her fertility as an adult. For instance, depending on the type of treatment, a girl treated for Hodgkin's disease before age fifteen has only about a 13 percent risk of permanent ovarian failure. From age fifteen to about age thirty, the risk is about 60 percent. Although some studies have found a very high risk of permanent menopause—nearly 100 percent—for women treated for Hodgkin's disease beyond age thirty, more current treatment regimens appear to be improving these odds.[13]

It's different with radiation—here, the younger a girl is, the more vulnerable she is to damage, because the uterus has not yet fully developed. Girls who haven't yet gone through puberty are more likely to have their uterus permanently damaged by radiation.

Just like with adult males, chemotherapy can damage boys' ability to produce sperm. It appears that boys who get chemotherapy prior to puberty have a better chance of recovering than those who get it after puberty, but they're vulnerable no matter what their age. Amazingly, though, some young men have recovered sperm production as many as fourteen years after cancer treatment.

Early Menopause

Even when fertility returns after chemotherapy and radiation, these treatments often lead to early menopause. So if you finished chemo and radiation at age thirty, and all the parts seem to be working fine now, don't assume that your "fertile window" is the same as that of your cancer-free friends. Odds are that you will enter menopause earlier than you otherwise would have. Just how much earlier, no one can say. Most doctors will tell you that, to get a crystal-ball look at how old you'll be when you hit menopause, look at how old your mom was when *she* did. (An exception: if your mom was a regular smoker and you're not, or vice versa, she's not a good predictor for you anymore. Yep, cigarette smoking has that much of an effect on ovarian function.) So, if your mom went into menopause at forty-five, take a few years off that figure for the effects of chemotherapy and radiation. You'll want to think about that when you start figuring out *when* you should try to conceive.

What You Can Do

After this litany of all the things that cancer and cancer treatment can do to lay waste to your body and leave you unable to have a baby, you might be even more depressed than when you picked up this book. But don't stop reading, because from now on, we're going to be talking about the good stuff.

Here's a little-known secret: almost everyone who's undergone treatment for cancer as a younger person can still find a way to be a parent. Whatever route you take, it probably won't be easy. The process can be infuriating and frustrating and seem like insult added to very serious illness if you're watching all of your friends start or add to their families at the same time you're tossing your cookies in the toilet, peeing orange from the latest round of chemotherapy, and getting ultrasounds to check for metastases rather than to find out the gender of a growing baby.

But *it can be done*. And let's face it—is there anything about being a parent that's ever easy? Plus, we've had cancer: we already know about fighting uphill battles against difficult odds. Don't tell us we can't do it.

First, your chances of conceiving spontaneously after chemotherapy, radiation, surgery, or other treatments might be better than you think. I figured that there was no way in the world I could get pregnant at age forty, after being slammed with chemotherapy at thirty-seven. But we conceived my son the first month we started trying. (With my younger daughter, it took two months.) We were far from alone. At a recent follow-up visit, my oncologist had just come from meeting with another patient who was thirty-seven weeks pregnant and had conceived without any assistance, several years after being treated for breast cancer.

There is also an ever-growing array of options for preserving your fertility before and during treatments and for assisting with conceiving a child afterward. Some of them are well known and reliable and some are still experimental, but you have more choices than ever before—you just have to know about them!

Even if pregnancy is not a possibility for you or your partner, adoption can be. You might be afraid that an expectant mother considering adoption would never pick you as a cancer survivor or that no country would ever approve you for international adoption—but a lot of the time, you'd be wrong.

And we're not done yet. There's also surrogacy, embryo adoption and donation, and foster care. We'll talk about all of these different paths to parenthood in the next few chapters. So no matter what treatment you're about to face, or how cancer may have ravaged your reproductive capabilities, if you have love to give to a child, you can find a way or make one. The rest of this book will tell you how.

CHAPTER 2

Hold On to What You've Got

Fertility Preservation

MY ONCOLOGIST WAS ONE of the good ones. When I was diagnosed with breast cancer, as a newlywed just a few weeks away from my first anniversary and my thirty-seventh birthday, she made sure to talk about fertility with my husband and me. (As I mentioned in the previous chapter, many oncologists still don't do that, although they're getting better.)

She explained that, before starting chemotherapy, I could go through a process to retrieve eggs and freeze either the eggs themselves or embryos fertilized with my husband's sperm. My first reaction: "You've got to be kidding me! I've just been promised that the next nine months of my life will be an endless round of drugs, doctors, surgeries, and tests, and now I'm supposed to sign on for more needles, more tests, more poking and prodding and procedures?"

Well, yes.

Ultimately, I decided to forego fertility preservation options and more or less roll the dice with my (already aging) ovaries. But no matter what your age, if you want to take active measures to protect your fertility and improve your chances of being able to bear or father children when you come out the other side of the cancer tunnel, you're going to have to add a little something extra to all the fun and games you're going through with your cancer specialists.

For Men

Let's start with fertility preservation for men because it's usually short and simple: banking sperm. If you're an adult male, unless your cancer has already depleted your sperm production (some do), there's pretty much no reason you can't walk into the appropriate facility, grab a few magazines or videos and a cup, and come out a while later with your reproductive future reasonably well protected. (You can find sperm banks, also called *cryobanks*, through online directories like www.spermbankdirectory.com.) It's not exactly romantic, but it's uncomplicated and noninvasive.

It also doesn't operate on the same schedule as a woman's menstrual cycle. A man doesn't have to wait until a magic time of the month to bank sperm. It's best if you haven't had sex within forty-eight hours of banking sperm, because it takes some time to replenish sperm levels after each ejaculation. But if you don't even have that much time to wait, experts say that twenty-four hours after ejaculation is usually enough to get a sufficient volume of semen. (It's also best to make at least two "deposits," separated by twenty-four to forty-eight hours, if you can.)

So even if you've been diagnosed with an advanced or fast-moving cancer that requires you to start treatment like, yesterday, if you're committed to having biological kids someday, you can squeeze in an appointment to retrieve sperm. Cycling legend Lance Armstrong was in a bad way by the time he got his diagnosis of testicular cancer that had spread to his lungs, abdomen, and brain—but even with the clock ticking, he had time to bank the sperm that eventually became son Luke and twin daughters Isabella and Grace.

Unfortunately, not all states have cryobank facilities. According to the Lance Armstrong Foundation (LAF), as of late 2009, six states—Alaska, Delaware, New Hampshire, Rhode Island, Vermont, and Wyoming—had no sperm banks at all, and other states might only have one or two that aren't easy for men on the other side of the state to get to.

But there's even a solution to that: you can bank sperm by mail. The LAF and Fertile Hope, a national nonprofit focused on fertility for cancer survivors (now a part of LAF), recently created LIVE:ON, a program that allows men to collect and bank sperm using at-home kits. You can either order a kit for free directly from their partner, Cryogenic Laboratories, Inc. (CLI), at www.liveonkit.com, or get one from your cancer center. When you return the kit to CLI, you're charged a $675 fee that includes processing, analysis (such as testing for infectious diseases like HIV and hepatitis B, as well as assessing the quality and motility of the sperm), freezing, and one year's storage. When you're ready to use the sperm, CLI will send the frozen samples to your reproductive endocrinologist. You may not get a sample that is quite as high quality as you'd get in an actual sperm banking facility, but it's still an effective procedure and a much better alternative to not banking sperm at all.

Men who bank sperm, if they're not married now, will someday have to explain to a partner that their only option for biological children together involves some form of artificial insemination—either *in vitro fertilization*, in which eggs are retrieved from the woman and fertilized with the man's sperm in the lab before being returned to the uterus, or *intrauterine insemination*, in which the sperm are simply injected into the uterus using a catheter.

Scott Greenberg found himself in that position. He had been diagnosed with stage II Hodgkin's disease in 1992, just after he started film school at NYU. He banked sperm. "My parents were quite nervous about telling me about the option, but someone else already had," he recalls. "My friends teased me and told me I should tear out pages of the magazines I'd looked at so I could show my future kids who their 'real mother' was. It was a relief to have that option, because getting married and having kids one day was a huge part of my life." But six years later, when Scott married his wife, Rachel, the conversation changed. Rachel had been adopted and was very open to the idea of adoption herself. "Still, I'd gone to such great lengths to freeze my sperm, we thought we should try to 'continue my bloodline.'"

Scott and Rachel went through several half-humorous, half-stressful cycles of intrauterine insemination, but a few months later, she wasn't getting pregnant. "We couldn't be the typical couple having a few problems; there's a finite amount of sperm here. I'd saved up quite a bit over a few weeks, but we wanted to have multiple kids," he says. "And the fertility treatments were getting so stressful, especially for my wife—it was affecting her weight, and she's an actress and she doesn't need that happening. She has a needle phobia and I had to stab her in the ass with the meds. For us it felt so unnatural, and she wasn't taking well to it." So Scott and Rachel eventually decided to pursue domestic adoption. We'll revisit them in chapter 5 to see how it went.

Jim DeLaere had a very different experience. He and his wife, Joy, had been married for two-and-a-half years when he was diagnosed with testicular cancer in October 2001. He had one testicle removed surgically, and doctors told the couple they had a small window of time to try to get pregnant. They weren't successful, and the day after Thanksgiving, Jim and Joy found out the cancer had gone to his blood and he would have to begin four rounds of chemotherapy by the middle of December.

Jim, a technical director for the couple's Illinois church, banked sperm before starting chemo. Two years after his successful treatment, with no sign of the cancer's recurring, the couple decided to start trying for a family. "We had pretty strong opinions going into it about the ethics of fertilizing embryos, and we wanted to only fertilize three eggs," says Joy, a freelance writer. "Because Jim had banked sperm, we had only six samples to use. Once they thaw a sample they have to use it right away, so we were told it would be wisest to do in vitro since it had a higher success rate."

After a couple of negative experiences at other fertility centers, Jim and Joy ended up at the Fertility Centers of Illinois in March 2004. "Quickly, they got me into the first IVF cycle—I'd had a lot of tests done already," Joy says. "We started drugs in April, and I had egg retrieval in the middle of May. We fertilized three eggs, got two embryos and put them both in, and found out in June that we were pregnant with one." On March 10, 2005, Jim and Joy's daughter Lillian was born. "We couldn't believe how easily it had gone! We knew a lot of people who had failed."

When they were ready for a second child, Jim and Joy figured they had gotten lucky the first time and should start trying early, since it might take them a while to conceive again. "No one told me that once you've successfully completed one IVF cycle, it's more likely to happen again!" says Joy. They returned to their doctor when Lillian was just eleven months old, and six weeks later, Joy was pregnant again. Their son Lincoln was born in November 2006. But when they failed in their attempt to conceive a third child through IVF, Jim and Joy decided to try to adopt from foster care—a journey you'll read more about in chapter 5.

Other Options for Men

What if it appears that you don't have any viable sperm, or any sperm at all—either before or after cancer treatment? Just because they can't find any sperm present in your semen doesn't mean that you don't have any at all. There might still be sperm in your testicular tissue that can be extracted and used with in vitro fertilization to get your partner pregnant.

Testicular sperm extraction is an outpatient procedure; basically, the doctors biopsy some tissue from your testicles and examine it for sperm cells. If they find any—which happens up to 45 percent of the time in cancer survivors—they can be removed and either used immediately or frozen for later use.

This isn't quite as easy as sperm banking, of course. But on the plus side, it can be done either before or after cancer treatment. (Remember that some men with testicular and other cancers may find that they already have very low sperm counts even before chemotherapy and radiation.)

Surgery for testicular cancer usually involves the removal of one or both testicles (orchiectomy). If only one testicle is cancerous, you'll still have one remaining to produce sperm. But what if both are cancerous? It may be possible to remove only part of one or both of the testicles, which could preserve some hormone and sperm production. This is called a partial orchiectomy. Ask your doctor if this could be a possibility for you.

If you've been diagnosed with early-stage (stage I) testicular cancer, you may also have another fertility-sparing option: a surgical approach known as nerve-sparing retroperitoneal lymph node dissection (RPLND). One of the side effects of surgery done to remove potentially cancerous lymph nodes in the retroperitoneum is something called "retrograde ejaculation"—when the man ejaculates, the sperm travels into the bladder instead of out the opening of the penis. This isn't harmful—except, of course, if you're trying to get someone pregnant. Nerve-sparing RPLND, although a more complex surgery, can help to prevent retrograde ejaculation; in addition, choosing to have these lymph nodes removed also permits some men to avoid chemotherapy altogether, eliminating *that* danger to their fertility.[1]

But keep in mind that even if you *do* have retrograde ejaculation due to surgery for testicular cancer, that doesn't mean you don't still have sperm in your ejaculate. Sometimes certain medications can, at least temporarily, correct retrograde ejaculation caused by nerve damage. If that doesn't work for you, sperm *can* be collected from the urine—although expertise is needed to do this so that the sperm will survive their time in this relatively hostile environment—and then used to fertilize your partner's eggs in traditional assisted reproduction methods such as in vitro fertilization (IVF).

For Women

If you're a woman, preserving your fertility through cancer treatment is a lot more complicated and usually more invasive. (Isn't that always the way?) You can't just walk into an "egg banking" facility and stroll out an hour later with a dozen eggs happily stored for posterity.

Still, you do have a number of options to consider—some of them well tested and proven successful and others still experimental. To some extent, your choices will depend on the type of cancer you have and how urgent the need to begin treatment is. But ultimately, what type of fertility preservation you choose—or if you choose none at all, as many women do—will depend primarily on *you*. How do you see yourself becoming a parent? Do you have a partner? What are your religious beliefs? How would you feel about having frozen embryos that you ended up not using?

Embryo Freezing

If your oncologist talks to you about fertility preservation, probably the first option you'll hear about is embryo freezing. That's because it has the longest and best track record of success. If you want a "take-home baby," embryo freezing gives you the best odds. Success rates range from 19 to 30 percent—which actually compares pretty well to the odds the average couple has of conceiving spontaneously in any given month. Hundreds of thousands of babies have been born around the world using this technique.

Your personal odds of success may vary from the averages, of course. Like everything else with a woman's fertility, the most important factor in the success of embryo freezing is how old you are when you retrieve the eggs. If you're thirty-five or younger when you retrieve eggs, fertilize them, and freeze the embryos, your overall chances of at least one successful pregnancy—no matter how old you are when you come back and implant them— are about 40 percent, according to Dr. Chung of the University of Southern California. That's because the uterus doesn't age the way that eggs do; your "biological clock" ticks loudest in your ovaries, not your uterus.

If you're between thirty-five and forty when you retrieve eggs and freeze embryos, your odds of eventual pregnancy are lower— about 30 percent, says Dr. Chung. That's because older eggs mean fewer viable embryos.

What does embryo freezing involve? For you, the patient, and your partner, it's pretty much the same process that you'd face if you were struggling with plain old ordinary everyday infertility (as opposed to the possibility of extra-special, super-charged, lemon-freshened, cancer-related infertility) and decided to undergo in vitro fertilization.

First, you wait for your period to start. Yes, I said wait. When you're diagnosed with cancer, the last thing you think you have is time. The idea of waiting to do anything is terrifying. But as my social worker at Sloan-Kettering told me, most cancers are immediate emotional emergencies—*not* immediate medical emergencies. This means that, in most cases (although not all the time—such as with fast-moving blood cancers like leukemia and Hodgkin's disease), you have a few weeks to meet with doctors, get second opinions, and, if you want, preserve your fertility.

And in fact, fertility preservation doesn't necessarily delay treatment at all. A recent Stanford University study of young women with breast cancer found that the median time from diagnosis to the start of chemotherapy was only four days longer in women who sought fertility preservation than in those who didn't (seventy-one vs. sixty-seven days).[2]

So, you wait for your period to start. Then, for about ten to twelve days, you inject yourself with hormones designed to stimulate egg development. (During most menstrual cycles, your body releases only one egg—when you're trying to retrieve eggs for embryo freezing, you need more than that!) Many women with cancers that are fed by hormones worry that using the same hormones to stimulate ovulation might also fuel the fire of their cancer. Although it's unclear whether this is true or not, your reproductive endocrinologist can customize your egg-stimulating regimen to minimize risk. Dr. Kutluk Oktay has published research showing that you can use letrozole (Femara) in combination with follicle-stimulating drugs to kick-start ovulation without significantly increasing worrisome hormone levels.[3] A side benefit: it's also about a thousand dollars cheaper than the usual course of hormones.

You'll get regular ultrasounds and blood work to monitor the eggs' growth, and once the eggs are mature, they'll be removed in a short outpatient surgical procedure (about twenty minutes) under light anesthesia. On the day of the extraction, your partner will also be asked to produce sperm for fertilization; the resulting embryos are then frozen and stored.

Jennifer Bolstad remembers the process vividly. She was thirty-two and married for less than three years when she was diagnosed with breast cancer in August 2008. "I found the lump myself. I had lost an aunt to breast cancer in her thirties, but it still never occurred to me that it could happen to me. It was this giant shock, even though maybe it shouldn't have been," she says. "And then I thought, wow! What am I going to do about having kids?"

Jennifer's biopsy results came back on August 4, and by August 8, she was sitting in Dr. Oktay's office. "He told me, you're on the right day of your cycle, so you need to start hormones now. There aren't any words to describe it; it's like you just go into survival mode. You're making decisions like, not the same way that you would if you had a long time to think about it. You feel like you have an infinitely long time to think about having children until you're sitting in a doctor's office and he says it's now or never, you're on day two of your cycle. Do I want to have children? Yes I do. I'm not taking any chances."

The first drug Jennifer took was letrozole (Femara), mentioned above. "A couple of days later, I started injections of a drug called Follistim—which does exactly what it sounds like," Jennifer says. "All the while I was going in for ultrasounds and blood draws every day or two. I'd never been aware of my ovaries as a body part before. It was like, oh my God, they're like giant footballs! They were very, very heavy." When the eggs were ready, Jennifer received a *Lupron trigger*—an injection of a drug that causes the eggs to release all at once.

The outpatient egg retrieval wasn't as easy as Jennifer expected. "There were only two times during the whole cancer treatment process that I was like, help me, Jesus—and one was after the egg retrieval," she recalls. "I felt really lousy afterward, the worst cramps of my life. But it could have also been everything else going on—I was doing PET scans, CT scans, test after test, and I knew I was starting chemo two days later."

Today, Jennifer and her husband are still waiting to try to get pregnant. After concluding chemotherapy, surgery, and radiation, she's on a three-year trial of the drug Zometa (zoledronic acid) for early-stage breast cancer and wants to finish out the trial first.

"When I sat down with my oncologist after the egg retrieval, she said, 'You just bought yourself a really expensive insurance policy. You're thirty-two years old, and chances are that when all is said and done, you're going to be able to have children the old-fashioned way.' Even hearing her say that, I'm very, very happy that I have those fourteen embryos in the bank."

Courtney Bugler was twenty-eight when she was diagnosed with breast cancer in October 2005. Because she and her husband were already trying to get pregnant, she had "babies on the brain" and immediately asked about fertility preservation. After her lumpectomy, Courtney did one egg retrieval cycle and, to her surprise, harvested thirty-four eggs. Of those, eighteen were fertilized with her husband's sperm and waited in storage while Courtney completed chemotherapy and radiation and moved from Illinois, where she'd been a television writer, to Atlanta, where she became executive director of the local branch of the Young Survival Coalition, a leading organization for young women with breast cancer.

After two years on Tamoxifen, Courtney's doctors told her she could "take a break" and try to get pregnant if she wanted. Her menstrual cycle had come back after chemotherapy, so there was no reason to think it wouldn't return again if she stopped Tamoxifen. "But the doctors argued that I could get pregnant and have the baby faster by in vitro rather than trying to conceive spontaneously, which would mean I could then get back on Tamoxifen faster."

Courtney also took the more unusual step of having an oophorectomy (removing her ovaries) before getting pregnant. "Some research shows that removing estrogen is good for preventing a cancer recurrence, and I knew I wouldn't be needing my ovaries, so I felt better that if I wouldn't be on Tamoxifen, I'd at least be doing something."

With the first IVF cycle using the frozen embryos, Bugler got pregnant but miscarried at eight weeks. "I spent a couple of weeks after that in full-on depression in a way I hadn't been with cancer," she said. "I felt like my body had done nothing but fail me for years."

But it didn't fail her the second time. After waiting a month, they tried again, and this time the pregnancy stuck. "Everything was delightful and normal. I liked being normal. I felt fine, I traveled at thirty-six weeks, and worked until 10:30 the night before I had the baby."

Courtney's son Aidan was born in August 2009, and by the time he was five months old, weighed twenty pounds. "He's a small pony," she says proudly. "He's as adorable as every parent thinks their child is."

Egg Freezing

Freezing eggs, not embryos, is becoming more common for women diagnosed with cancer. You might consider egg freezing instead of embryo freezing if you don't have a partner right now and aren't comfortable with the idea of using donor sperm, or if you have religious or ethical concerns about freezing and storing embryos given that you might not have the opportunity to implant them all later.

Egg freezing is a newer technique than embryo freezing, and it's still considered experimental. As of 2009, about nine hundred babies had been born via egg freezing, most within the last few years.

Eggs are a lot harder to freeze than embryos—they're large cells that contain a lot of water, so ice crystals can form during the freezing process. "Eggs also have all these very fragile components that need to be functional to produce a chromosomally normal embryo," says USC's Dr. Chung. "Ice crystals forming in a frozen egg can cause irreparable chromosomal damage."

Within the last several years, there have been some significant advances in egg freezing. There are two main approaches: *fast freezing* (vitrification) and *slow freezing* (controlled-rate freezing). Some researchers think vitrification is better, but Dr. Chung believes that the important element in either technique is how you use *cryoprotectants*—a fancy word for antifreeze. "We need cryoprotectants, but they're also thought to be potentially toxic, and you want to reduce exposure," she says. "By playing around with the way we employ cryoprotectants, it's helped us to freeze eggs better."

Egg-freezing technology was so new that USC didn't think it was responsible to offer to patients until about five years ago. "Since then, we've started seeing more patients and offering it as an alternative, with the understanding that it's investigational," Dr. Chung says. "We've had a number of women here for cancer treatment come in and freeze eggs, but no one has come back to use them yet. Ultimately, though, I think that egg freezing will work as well as embryo freezing. For young girls who don't want to commit genetically to a sperm donor, egg freezing is a viable option for them."

"All indications are that the gap between egg and embryo freezing is closing," agrees Dr. Oktay. "Our experience is increasing, and just like what happened with IVF, more and more pregnancies are happening. Right now, the success rate is about 50 percent of what you get with embryo freezing. I think that will get better with time."

The process for having your eggs frozen is exactly like having embryos frozen—you just skip the step at the end where you have a partner providing a sperm donation to fertilize the eggs with. Instead, the eggs are immediately frozen instead of being fertilized.

That's what Lindsay Nohr Beck did. The founder of Fertile Hope, and one of the first cancer patients to freeze eggs, Lindsay immediately thought about kids when she was diagnosed with tongue cancer at the age of twenty-two. "We were talking about my tongue, so my mind went to eating, speaking, kissing—and then to marriage and kids." Doctors assured her that her treatment, radiation to the head and neck, would not affect her future fertility.

But eighteen months later, the cancer had returned and spread to her neck. This time, Lindsay needed surgery and chemotherapy as well as radiation. Doctors told her that there was a very high risk that she could become permanently infertile. This was in 2000, when the worlds of cancer and fertility treatment had not yet come together, so they had no options to offer her. "I said, my hair will grow back and I won't puke for the rest of my life, but infertility is not an option," Lindsay says. "I had a window of six to eight weeks between surgery and starting chemo, so while I was healing from having part of my tongue removed, I was calling people trying to figure out my reproductive options. I figured, men can bank sperm; I'll bank eggs."

It wasn't that easy. Fertility centers all told her that they only banked embryos, not eggs. But Lindsay wasn't married or seriously dating, and she just couldn't envision fertilizing eggs with donor sperm and then, ten years down the road, telling her future husband that she could be biologically related to their children, but he couldn't be. "I didn't want to impose this random third-party sperm on us," she says.

After hundreds of calls, Lindsay happened to reach a doctor at Stanford who told her that they'd just started an egg-freezing program for cancer patients, and she could come in the next day. "It all fell into place with my cycle, and twelve days later I had twenty-nine eggs frozen. They warned me that the success rates were like 2 to 3 percent per egg, but I said, that's better than zero.

And I don't need them today—I'll need them down the road, and hopefully by then technology will improve."

Perhaps surprisingly, Lindsay says that the actual process of freezing her eggs was "the best experience ever." That's because, in contrast to the everyday doctor's appointments and twice-a-day radiation she was then undergoing, the "egg appointments" felt like planning for the future. "Everybody involved in egg freezing believed I would survive," she says. "It was so positive, so hopeful, so tangible. Having done that helped me sit through chemo and accept that poison into my body."

But isn't fertility treatment a roller coaster for most couples? Lindsay thinks there's a big difference between preserving fertility and trying to get pregnant. "Preserving fertility is short, fast, and successful. You bank sperm or freeze eggs or embryos, it takes two to four weeks at most, and you're done," she says. "You can feel a sense of hope. The roller coaster comes later, when you're trying to conceive. And that's something I went through down the road. But preserving fertility, for me, was a clear, easy plan that helped me get through cancer treatment."

Ultimately, Lindsay's cycles returned after chemotherapy, and when she met and married her husband, Jordan, doctors told her she should try to conceive on her own first, while she still had a window of fertility. (Even when your cycles do come back, chemotherapy on average takes about five to ten years off a woman's "fertile lifespan.")

It proved harder than expected. Lindsay's husband had a chromosomal problem called a balanced translocation, which causes miscarriages and severe chromosomal abnormalities in a certain percentage of pregnancies. Lindsay had six miscarriages before they figured out the problem and pursued in vitro fertilization using preimplantation genetic diagnosis (that is, the fertilized embryos would be tested for abnormalities before implantation). "The first cycle, we got twenty eggs and eighteen embryos, and all of them were bad. The next time, we had two normal embryos, transferred them both, and one turned into my daughter, Paisley," Lindsay says.

Lindsay has always wanted a big family and says she definitely plans on more kids. "I don't regret freezing the eggs—the cost, the time, any of it. I still may need them, and you make the best decision you can with the information you have at the time. The regret factor would've been so much higher if things were the opposite," she says. "It's like insurance. It's peace of mind. I'm not driving around saying, gee, I wish I'd get into a car accident and put my auto insurance to use."

Eggs or Embryos—or Both?

Embryo freezing and egg freezing are, at least for the moment, the two most common ways that young women with cancer choose to preserve their fertility. So how do you choose whether or not to freeze eggs or embryos?

A lot of the decision depends on whether or not you're married or in a very serious relationship. Most women who are in a committed relationship choose to freeze embryos since they know the man they want to have children with and embryo freezing is a more tested technology.

Women who are single, or in less committed relationships, are more likely to choose egg freezing, for the same reasons Lindsay Nohr Beck did. They can't imagine marrying the man of their dreams someday and saying, "Guess what? If I'm going to have biological kids, they're going to be fathered by someone else."

Some religious faiths may also have very specific concerns about IVF techniques, and that may play into your decision. Do you have trouble reconciling the idea of freezing embryos—some of which you may never be able to use—with your religious beliefs? If so, freezing unfertilized eggs that you can fertilize only when you know you're ready to try to conceive may be a better choice for you.

These are tough choices. "Some young women who aren't married have opted for a good friend, or a relationship that seems like it's going somewhere, to fertilize embryos for them," says Gwendolyn Quinn, PhD, of the H. Lee Moffitt Cancer Center and Research Institute in Tampa, Florida.[4] "That has caused some issues down the road. People who face infertility without a cancer diagnosis usually have at least a year to think about how they feel about all this, while people with cancer sometimes have four or five days, or less, to make their decisions. I know a couple of women three or four years out from embryo freezing who are very conflicted. In one case, the woman is no longer in the relationship with the man she used to create her embryos. Legally, she owns them, but she doesn't have good feelings toward him—yet her only chance to have a biological child is through his DNA."

Another possibility: should you cover all your bases and do both? At first glance, that might seem to make the most sense. After all, even if you're married now, no one knows the future. You might get divorced, become widowed, get remarried—possibilities that no one likes to think about, but if one of those things were to happen, what would you do if you only had frozen embryos? If you got divorced, would you still want to bear your ex's biological children? And would he let you?

Rochelle Barnes's husband wouldn't. Within a month after being diagnosed with stage II breast cancer in 2006, at the age of thirty-two, Rochelle (name changed at her request) was in a fertility clinic harvesting eggs to fertilize and preserve. Already the mother of a young daughter, she very much wanted more children. "We were able to freeze fifteen embryos, and that made all the difference in the world to me. If you have embryos, it doesn't matter if you have ovaries or not, all you need is your uterus," she says. "I had all my ducks in a row and I was ready to fight."

But shortly after her cancer treatment ended, Rochelle's marriage started going downhill. She kept thinking things would get better—but they didn't. She sought family therapy, then a trial separation. The couple stayed married long enough so that Rochelle could get a full mastectomy using her husband's health insurance; then they divorced.

"At first he was [saying] that I could have the embryos, but then he met someone and he wanted to have more babies, and I don't think she was very happy with the idea," says Rochelle. "I wanted him to just relinquish his claim to parental rights and have no financial obligations. I just wanted the option to have another child. I argued for them in the divorce negotiations, and they wouldn't have any of it. If I had frozen eggs as well as embryos, I wouldn't be in this position."

Rochelle might have been successful at pursuing "double coverage," because she was able to harvest eighteen eggs—and egg and embryo freezing are both a numbers game. The more you have, the better. "You have a 50 percent greater chance of a successful pregnancy with frozen embryos as compared to eggs," says Dr. Oktay. "So if you are able to retrieve eggs in the double digits, it might be worth freezing some of both. Anything less than that, probably not. Since only half as many frozen eggs will survive as embryos will, maybe you should freeze two-thirds of your eggs, and fertilize the rest and freeze those embryos."

Someday in the not-so-distant future, you may not have to take the gamble on freezing eggs. In the fall of 2010, researchers at Brown University in Providence, Rhode Island, announced that they had created the world's first "artificial ovary"—a lab-created cell structure that mimics the environment of a real ovary, where immature eggs can mature outside the body.[5] By avoiding the freezing and thawing process, which is so hazardous to eggs because of their high water content, researchers hope that eggs matured this way will have a much better chance of survival and, ultimately, being fertilized and nurtured through a successful pregnancy. When it's ready for prime time (don't go knocking on the door at Brown just yet), an artificial ovary would also be a particularly good solution for pediatric cancer patients and for those whose treatment needs won't allow them to wait long enough to undergo the standard egg-stimulation process, which brings eggs to maturity quickly while still inside a woman's body.

Ovarian Tissue Freezing and Transplants

What if you don't have time to freeze eggs or embryos? Some cancers, like lymphomas and leukemias, require you to start treatment almost immediately. Marybeth Gerrity, PhD, until recently the executive director of the Oncofertility Consortium, recalls an eighteen-year-old girl who went to the emergency room because she was having trouble breathing. "She thought it was asthma, but it was a lymphoma so big it was pressing on her lung," Gerrity says. "She had to start chemotherapy almost immediately."[6]

When the clock is not only ticking but the alarm is going off, even the few weeks of a fertility cycle are too long to wait. In that case, you can consider ovarian tissue *cryopreservation* (freezing).

Ovarian tissue cryopreservation is even more experimental than egg freezing. In 2004, a Belgian woman became the first to have a baby using this procedure: six years after becoming infertile after treatment for stage IV Hodgkin's lymphoma, Ouarda Touirat had strips of preserved ovarian tissue reimplanted. Four months later, her menstrual cycle returned, and Touirat became pregnant with a baby girl she named Tamara.

Since then, as of this writing, there have been approximately fourteen pregnancies worldwide as a result of ovarian tissue transplantation, all but two of them spontaneous—meaning that the women needed no further intervention to get pregnant, other than having the strips of ovarian tissue reimplanted.

Sounds exciting—but it's more complicated than that. Despite Touirat's success, doctors are very leery of transplanting actual ovarian tissue back into a woman who's had a blood-borne cancer (like lymphoma or leukemia). "There's too great a risk of reseeding you with your own cancer," warns Gerrity. A study published in 2010 found that cancer cells in women with leukemias can, indeed, contaminate the ovaries.[7]

"Now, last week we saw a twenty-three-year-old woman with colon cancer who needed immediate treatment," Dr. Gerrity relays. "We took out one of her ovaries and froze it, and down the road, she'd be a good candidate for ovarian tissue transplant. Women with brain tumors would be good candidates as well."

In 2008, a Danish woman, Stinne Holm Bergholdt, gave birth to her second child after having ovarian tissue frozen and reimplanted following a bout with Ewing's sarcoma. Bergholdt had her first daughter after the transplant in 2007, with the help of mild ovarian stimulation, and assumed that she'd need to have an additional transplant to conceive again (she had preserved a total of thirteen strips of tissue, six of which were reimplanted initially). But when she went to see her fertility specialist again in January 2008, it turned out that she was already pregnant with a second daughter, who was born in late 2008. Bergholdt's case is exciting, but it's important to be realistic about the numbers. Still, the technology is advancing, and her success represents all-important hope for women and girls who may not be able to freeze embryos or eggs.

For women who are deemed too high-risk for ovarian tissue transplant, researchers are now exploring another possibility: removing an ovary, then isolating follicles and growing fertilizable eggs in the laboratory. Northwestern University is now leading the biggest national trial of this *very* experimental approach. "It's moving forward quickly," says Gerrity. "Now, it's not for everyone to try. If you're thirty-nine, the technology probably isn't going to move forward in time. But if you're sixteen? Oh yeah." If you want to inquire about participating in a trial of ovarian tissue cryopreservation, contact the Oncofertility Consortium (see Resources, page 181).

If you happen to have an identical twin sister, you may have one other option: an actual ovary transplant. Infertility pioneer Sherman Silber, MD, of the Infertility Center of St. Louis, has performed nine ovary transplants between identical twin sisters when one of them has undergone premature ovarian failure. One of them, Anna Heard, is a leukemia survivor who, with her sister Rachel, was adopted from Korea at the age of fourteen months. A few months after receiving her sister's healthy ovary, Heard's menstrual cycle returned, and shortly after that, she was pregnant. She miscarried twice, however, before becoming pregnant with a healthy boy who was born in January 2010.

"I'm very grateful to my sister," Heard says. "She had no hesitation when it came to donating bone marrow for my marrow transplant, but that saves a life. Doing this may have ultimately put her fertility at risk too. It was a big deal for her to do this for me."

Ovarian Suppression

Isn't there a simpler way to preserve fertility during chemotherapy? Couldn't you do something to protect your ovaries from the toxic effects of chemo without yanking them out of your body altogether? That would be ideal, but science isn't there yet.

For quite a few years, some doctors have advised women who want to protect their fertility to take the drug Lupron (leuprolide) during chemotherapy. Lupron shuts down ovarian function, and the theory has been that chemo drugs won't have as toxic an effect on cells at rest as they do on those that are rapidly dividing.

Unfortunately, that's not always the case. Alkylating agents, like cyclophosphamide, don't just attack rapidly dividing cells. They kill cells at any stage, even the primordial follicles. "They just push them to cell suicide," says Dr. Oktay. "The reserve follicles, which are what we're concerned about, are quiescent, so using hormonal ways to stop follicle development isn't possible. We need to look at ways to prevent cell suicide or DNA damage to the eggs."

So Lupron is falling out of favor among specialists in cancer and fertility, and the quest is on for a better drug to prevent egg loss. "If we could figure out a medical treatment, women could avoid all these procedures," says Dr. Oktay. One drug that's shown promise in animals is called S1P (sphingosine 1-phosphate), but odds are that it or any other such drugs won't be available, even in experimental trials, for another couple of years.

Another possibility might be the drug Gleevec, which has revolutionized the treatment of chronic myelogenous leukemia (CML). In a 2009 study, Italian researchers found that the chemotherapy drug cisplatin destroys eggs by damaging a particular enzyme, known as c-abl. Gleevec, they found, stopped the egg damage caused by cisplatin.[8] This research was done in mice, so it too is a long way from the clinic at this point. For example, researchers still have to make sure that giving Gleevec at the same time as cisplatin, or any other chemotherapy drug, doesn't interfere with the chemotherapy's ability to kill cancer cells while it's also protecting eggs. And then, of course, all of this has to be studied in humans.

So, in the meantime, should you take Lupron during chemo? "Most studies show no benefit to it," says Dr. Chung. "A few show some, but there are problems with some of those. But at the same time, it doesn't hurt anything. If you're in a bind and have no other option, you can take it—but you have to realize that there's a good chance it won't make a difference."

Some women have used Lupron during chemo, had their cycles return quickly, and successfully become pregnant—but there's no way to know whether that would have happened anyway.

Ovarian Transposition

Yep, this is exactly what it sounds like—moving your ovaries around to get them out of the line of fire, if your particular type of cancer requires that radiation be beamed directly at your pelvic area. Some cancers for which ovarian transposition has been used to preserve fertility during treatment include colorectal cancer, cervical cancer, and Hodgkin's disease.

Your doctor can surgically move ovaries higher up into your abdomen, away from the radiation field, to minimize the amount of damage done to them during treatment. Fortunately, the surgery can be done in a minimally invasive outpatient procedure. Even if your cancer requires a hysterectomy, if you can hold on to functioning ovaries, you can conceive a baby through IVF techniques and seek a gestational surrogate to carry the pregnancy (more on that in chapter 4).

"With cervical cancer in particular, radiation primarily is focused on the area of the vagina," says Dr. Chung. "If you can get the ovaries out of the pelvis and up into the abdomen, you can shield them from some of the damage. We've done that here a number of times, and it's been very successful."

It isn't a perfect solution—your ovaries may still get hit with some scattered radiation, and it's possible that the very act of moving the ovaries could damage their blood supply. Fertile Hope reports that the success rate with ovarian transposition—that is, returning back to normal menstrual cycles—is about 50 percent.

Radical Trachelectomy

This is a still-experimental surgical procedure designed to allow patients with certain types of invasive cervical cancer to keep their uterus while having the cervix removed. (Almost half of all cervical cancer diagnoses are in women forty-five and under.)

Usually, if you're diagnosed with invasive cervical cancer, your doctor will recommend a pretty comprehensive and intense surgical approach: a radical hysterectomy and salpingo-oophorectomy, which pretty much means taking out all your girl parts—ovaries, uterus, and cervix. A radical trachelectomy instead removes only the cervix, parametrium, surrounding lymph nodes, and upper 2 cm of the vagina, leaving the uterus intact.

Not all women with cervical cancer are candidates for radical trachelectomy. You should have

- A squamous cell carcinoma or adenocarcinoma

- A lesion smaller than 2 cm

- No evidence of lymph node involvement

- A clear MRI scan that rules out cancer spread

To date, about six hundred women worldwide have undergone radical trachelectomy. About half of them have tried to become pregnant, and 60 percent have successfully conceived and carried pregnancies to term. As of summer 2008, according to the MD Anderson Cancer Center in Houston, Texas, 204 babies had been born to women who'd undergone radical trachelectomy.

This course of action doesn't appear to increase your risk of the cancer returning: women who've had radical trachelectomies experience recurrence and death after recurrence at about the same rates (4 percent and 2 percent, respectively) as women who have standard radical hysterectomies.

Pregnancy after radical trachelectomy is no walk in the park, though. You must give birth by C-section and you do have a slightly higher risk of miscarriage than the average woman. And it doesn't always work out.

Michelle Whitlock was a month shy of her twenty-seventh birthday when she was diagnosed with stage IB1 cervical cancer in 2001. The tumor was in the upper part of her cervical canal, and she was told she'd have to have a radical hysterectomy. Then living in Maryland, Michelle went to the library of the National Institutes of Health where she read about radical trachelectomy, and she began an ultimately successful fight with her HMO to allow her to have the procedure.

Two years later, Michelle was living in Memphis. She went out to dinner with her boyfriend, thinking they were celebrating two years in remission, and was bowled over when he proposed marriage. Then she got home. "There was a blinking light on my answering machine, and my doctor's voice on the message just said, 'Call me.' The phone slipped out of my hand. I knew, just from hearing her voice, that my cancer was back. I'd just gotten engaged, I knew I wanted to have children, and now I had to have a radical hysterectomy!"

Ultimately, Michelle squeezed in time before the procedure to harvest eggs and freeze embryos with her fiance so she could later find a gestational surrogate to help her have a baby. You'll read more of her story in chapter 4.

Conservative Ovarian Surgery

If you've been diagnosed with ovarian cancer, most of the time, doctors will recommend the removal of both of your ovaries. But with stage I ovarian cancer, meaning that the disease is still confined to the ovaries, it might be possible to have only one ovary removed—if, that is, only one is cancerous. You'll have to be followed even more closely if you choose this approach to treatment, because ovarian cancer can be very aggressive. But the good news is that the five-year survival rate with stage I ovarian cancer is nearly 100 percent, even if just the one ovary is removed.

If you do choose to have just one ovary removed, that may allow you to become pregnant after treatment, and subsequent pregnancy does not increase the risk that your cancer will come back. In fact, pregnancy and breastfeeding decrease your risk of developing ovarian cancer in the first place, although there haven't been any studies to determine if that would also mean that a post-cancer pregnancy would guard against ovarian cancer returning.

Children and Adolescents

When it comes to children and adolescents diagnosed with cancer, the options are in some ways much the same and in other ways very different. Girls and boys who've hit puberty often can choose from more or less the same possibilities for fertility preservation that adults can. But while harvesting eggs from a fourteen-year-old girl may be the same procedure, medically speaking, as harvesting them from a thirty two-year-old woman, emotionally speaking the two procedures aren't even on the same planet. Even banking sperm is a whole different thing to a teenage boy than to a guy in his thirties.

"It's hard. I had one mother of a sixteen-year-old girl say to me that as soon as you hear your child has cancer, you think, 'My child's on fire. Get the water, put them out,'" says Gwendolyn Quinn, PhD, of the Moffitt Cancer Center in Florida. "You know you should be thinking about all these other things, but it's hard to wrap your head around tomorrow. You're thinking about today."

If you're reading this book, you might be a teenager with cancer, but the odds are a lot greater that you're the mom or dad of that teenager, so I'm going to talk mostly to you. It's hard to think about your child as a sexual being—especially when you're focused so intently on just keeping that child alive—but it's a conversation you need to have, with yourself, with your spouse or partner, and with your child as well.

It will be a hard conversation for you as a parent to have. It's probably even harder for your child to think about. "You're twelve, and do your mom and dad make this decision for you?" asks Marybeth Gerrity. "Then what if you're twenty-six and your eggs have been stored and you don't want them? What if you don't have the money to pay for storage—do mom and dad have to do that for the rest of their lives?"

Researchers who've studied how young people react to cancer find that their attitudes about fertility vary widely. "I've heard some say, 'Well, God will still give you babies,'" says Gerrity. Others are more certain that they know what they want. "I met a sixteen-year-old with a brain tumor who was absolutely sure she wanted to freeze her ovarian tissue. She said, 'We teenagers are going to change the world. I participate in every study.'"

And some teenagers can cope with yet more treatments while some can't. "There's a lot of individual variation in teens," says Gerrity. "Some are quite mature and can handle the idea of daily vaginal ultrasounds and injections on top of whatever cancer treatment they're having. Others are younger and maybe less mature, and they can't."

When Karyn Buxman's son David was a junior in college, he woke up one morning with a pain in his chest that turned out to be a fist-sized tumor. It was testicular cancer (it's a little-known fact that this type of cancer can appear in the testicles *or* the chest, abdomen, or pelvis). "The specialist made a whirlwind entrance and started throwing out information: the tests are conclusive, it's cancer, it's growing fast, it's very dangerous, and we have to begin treatment right away, it's going to make you very sick and miserable, but if you don't have it, you're going to die. It was like a bomb blowing up in the room."

The meeting with the specialist was on a Thursday; he told David that he would have to start chemotherapy that Monday. In the midst of all the deluge of information, Karyn, who had a nursing background, thought of something. "Would the chemotherapy make him sterile?" she asked. The doctor said, "Well, yes." Looking at David, he asked "Do you have any children?" An overwhelmed David said no. "Do you want to have any?"

"Um, I think so . . ." David said.

"Oh. Well, let me think about this a minute."

The specialist arranged for his nurse to set up an appointment for David the next day at a fertility clinic. Meanwhile, he handed David a pamphlet to read. "He came to me a little teary and said, 'I don't know why they're bothering. This says one visit isn't really going to be enough," Karyn recalls. "The pamphlet did say something to the effect that the more deposits you can make, the greater your chance of having children. So I went to the nurse's desk and picked up the phone and made an appointment at the fertility clinic on Monday before he started chemo."

Karyn found the whole experience very troubling. "Had David not had an advocate, and had I not had the knowledge I had, the whole situation might have turned out very differently," she says. "There's so much information being thrown at you, and as soon as you hear cancer, it's 'wah wah wah' like a Charlie Brown cartoon. You're so scared and confused and absorbing so little of the information."

When her daughter was diagnosed with a sarcoma at the age of sixteen, Timi Gleason went through exactly that kind of confusion and information overload. "I don't remember them talking to me about future fertility, if they did," she says. "But then shortly after she stopped chemo, they were doing blood work and something came up that there were problems with her eggs. We went to see a fertility doctor, and it turned out that her eggs and hormone levels were not where they should be for her age. I felt betrayed that we hadn't been told about this at first. We let Krissy make the decision about chemo, and I was relatively passive."

Today, tests show that Krissy's hormone levels may be heading in the right direction, but she tells her mother that it doesn't matter. "She said, 'It's not a big deal, I don't care.' I said, 'I wonder if that's really true. When you were a little girl you were going to have seventeen babies!' She told me that if she doesn't have kids, she'll just have a career, but I wonder if she'll always feel that way," Timi says. "But we just sort of trudge forward. That's how she and I are. We don't stop and get too romantic about stuff."

Before Puberty

If your daughter or son hasn't yet reached puberty, options for preserving their fertility are much more limited. Prepubescent boys can't bank sperm, and girls can't retrieve and freeze eggs. If they're undergoing pelvic radiation, both boys and girls can and should have as much shielding as possible to protect their reproductive organs, and girls have the option of undergoing ovarian transposition to protect their ovaries.

But beyond that, the only fertility preservation choices you have are ovarian tissue preservation for girls and testicular tissue freezing for boys. Keep in mind that both of these procedures are experimental; ovarian tissue transplants have resulted in a few pregnancies, but so far, testicular tissue freezing has not.

And while both of these procedures are minimally invasive, they're yet another surgery that a child facing cancer treatment must undergo. It's an agonizing choice to make: do you put your child through one more confusing, scary treatment in the hopes of preserving their chances of having children of their own later?

Beth Page elected not to. Her daughter, Tanner, was diagnosed with pre-B cell acute lymphocytic leukemia at age six and is now in the midst of a two-and a-half-year course of treatment that will involve chemotherapy—but no planned radiation. "Although I'm not naive enough to think the chemo couldn't or won't affect her ability to have kids, the radiation is the more known culprit for causing fertility issues and it is not included in Tanner's treatment plan," says Beth. "If she were a boy and a teenager, I might have considered freezing a sperm sample before treatment. But, as she is six and a girl, there's really nothing we can do about it, and as with many things, I table the things we cannot control and try to focus our efforts on getting our family through this whole and alive."

When Laurie Hanson's daughter Julie (name changed at her request) was first diagnosed with cancer at age eleven, she had not yet entered puberty. Like Tanner, she went through a grueling two-and a-half-year course of treatment that included some experimental chemotherapy, but no radiation. "I have a vague memory of talking about fertility a bit with the first treatment," Laurie says. "If that memory serves, they said something like fertility was a much bigger issue for males with that particular treatment and they weren't particularly concerned."

But a few years later, at age fourteen, Julie was diagnosed again—this time with myelodysplasia, which the doctors said was probably a result of all the chemotherapy she'd had the first time. This course of treatment included a bone marrow transplant— which would almost certainly devastate Julie's future fertility. "Before the transplant, it was a conversation of possibilities. Following up after the transplant, they verified with hormone testing that she had in fact, lost her fertility," says Laurie. "They said to continue using birth control no matter what if you don't want to have a child, because there's always a slim possibility of conceiving, but the likelihood was almost zero. She is on a lifetime course of the Pill just to replace the estrogen that she's not producing for herself."

Although the doctors did briefly discuss the possibility of harvesting eggs, which was a possibility because Julie had begun to menstruate by then, they didn't recommend it. The technology, at the time, was even more experimental than it is today (Julie's now a sophomore in college). "The message was clear: it was such an invasive procedure, and she'd been through so much already," says Laurie. "She wasn't interested, and we didn't push it."

Laurie still remembers talking with Julie about her options for having children in the future. "I told her that when she was born, I just kind of had this epiphany that it really did not matter how she arrived in my life. I was going to love whatever child came my way to be in my care, and when she was born I really had the understanding that adoption was an equally wonderful way to have a child come into your life," she recalls. "It comes up every now and then; she'll let me know that she's looking at or thinking about the ethnicity of her future children—what kind of family she'd like to create. She's in a good place, so far."

Laurie's advice for other parents grappling with these decisions: "Do your best to separate your own interests from your child's interests, and think about the price your child may have to pay either way."

Costs and Coverage

So how much do all these complicated procedures cost? It varies widely. In most cases, ovarian transposition, radical trachelectomy, and even Lupron injections are considered part of your course of cancer treatment and are covered by insurance (if you have it) with few to no hitches. And since ovarian tissue cryopreservation is such an experimental procedure, you can often have all or most of your costs covered by participating in a supervised clinical trial.

Embryo and egg freezing are another matter. As anyone who's gone through fertility treatments of any kind knows, they're *expensive*—and while many insurance plans do pay for them, many others don't, and those that do often have strict rules about how much they will cover.

In general, according to Fertile Hope, the average cost of embryo freezing and IVF is about $10,000 per cycle, with medications running an additional $2,000 to $5,000. Egg freezing is a little cheaper—an average of about $8,000 with the same additional costs for medications. Sperm banking, on average, costs about $1,500 for extraction plus five years of storage. Testicular sperm extraction costs vary widely, ranging from $6,000 to $16,000.

So how are you going to pay for all this? If you have insurance coverage, you might be surprised at how much you can convince your carrier to pay for, if you take the right approach. If you don't, or if they don't cover everything, there are other paths you can take.

Dealing with Insurance Companies

First, don't think of yourself as a fertility patient. Think of yourself as a *cancer* patient for whom infertility is a *known side effect of treatment*. If you have insurance, that's the way you need to get your insurance carrier to look at your situation in order to get as much coverage as possible.

"Your doctors need to be using accurate codes when they bill—not fertility codes, which most fertility providers are trained to use, but cancer diagnosis codes along with fertility preservation codes," says Gerrity. "We've been very successful in getting our patients insurance coverage on a case-by-case basis. You may have to jump through a few hoops or appeal, but a lot of people have to do that with their insurance for all kinds of reasons these days."

The Oncofertility Consortium provides sample letters of medical necessity and appeal for your doctors to use in seeking coverage from your insurer. These are reproduced at the end of this chapter with permission. What's key: the letter needs to mention that your potential infertility is a *known* side effect of a *covered treatment* and that the fertility preservation technique you plan to use is the *standard of care* for patients in your given situation.

"Two weeks ago, I saw a patient who had testicular cancer years ago and now wanted to use IVF to father a child," says Gerrity. "He had his doctor use our letters and got the insurance company to pay for up to three cycles to achieve a first pregnancy—in a state with no mandated coverage for infertility and with an insurer that usually doesn't cover fertility treatments."

If you and your doctor can't convince your insurer to cover the fertility preservation technique you both believe is best for you, you can contact the Oncofertility Consortium (see Resources, page 181) and ask for their advice.

Sharing Hope

If your income levels meet certain criteria (generally $50,000 or less for an individual, or $75,000 or less for a household), you can often get funding assistance for certain aspects of fertility preservation from Fertile Hope's Sharing Hope program. Sharing Hope supports

- Access to sperm banking (covering sperm extraction, analysis, and a year of storage)
- Discounted rates on one cycle of embryo or egg freezing, through partnerships with specific physicians and centers
- Free or reduced-cost fertility medications

Other Financial Options

Some cancer centers have been able to negotiate reduced-cost fertility preservation services for their patients. "Our fertility program doesn't charge a consultation fee to our patients, and they offer reduced fees and a payment plan and participate in Sharing Hope," says Gwendolyn Quinn. Ask your provider if they have anything like this for their patients—or if they'd be willing to try to negotiate for you.

If you know that there are expenses associated with your fertility preservation that your insurance won't cover, you can save at least some of the cost by contributing pretax dollars to a health savings account. You can set one up with a bank, a credit union, or an insurance company; many employers offer this option as well. Pretax dollars contributed to a health savings account can be used to pay for a surprising number of fertility-related expenses that may not be covered by your insurance, including everything from IVF and other fertility treatments for yourself, your spouse, or a dependent (but not for a surrogate), down to pregnancy tests and those over-the-counter fertility monitors you see in the drugstore.

If you own your home, you might also consider a Home Equity Line of Credit (HELOC) to help finance fertility preservation treatments. The interest on the loan is tax deductible, and you can usually write checks on the loan for just the amount you need. For example, if you're approved for a $20,000 HELOC, you can pay your individual bills using the loan rather than taking the whole amount out in one lump sum.

What's Right for You?

Now that you've read about all your options, your head is probably spinning with new terminology and images of various surgical procedures, hormone injections, and medications. How do you weigh your choices? How do you decide which of the possibilities is right for you?

In some cases, the decision may be made *for* you, by the speed with which your cancer is advancing, by what your insurance company will cover, or by what is available to you at the center where you're being treated or anywhere within a reasonable travel distance. Or perhaps it's just the only appropriate procedure for your particular type of cancer.

But a lot of people with cancer—women, especially—will have to make a choice: Egg freezing? Embryo freezing? A combination of both? Ovarian tissue freezing or some other type of surgery? Do nothing and hope that you'll get lucky?

No two people, even given the exact same circumstances, will make the same choice. Even when it seems obvious, it may not be. Lindsay Beck, in her twenties, could probably have thrown caution to the wind and not frozen eggs. Most women under thirty who undergo standard chemotherapy will retain their fertility, even if they might end up hitting menopause a little earlier than usual. But she wanted that "insurance policy."

Meanwhile, I was thirty-seven, married, and had been about to start trying to get pregnant literally the month I was diagnosed with breast cancer. Since I was approaching that doomsday deadline of forty, it would have made the most sense for me to freeze embryos. But I didn't. It wasn't because I wasn't given the information. I just decided that I couldn't cope with the idea of another battery of tests, procedures, drugs, and needles right before I jumped on the cancer treatment merry-go-round for an ugly eight-month whirl. I knew that meant I might be sacrificing my chance to have biological children forever, and I struggled some with that—my husband even more than I did—but ultimately, fertility preservation just didn't feel right for me.

Lindsay and I both made the right decisions for us, even though they might seem like the complete opposite of the choices you'd expect us to make. And that's the key. Only you know what's most important for you, what your priorities are about having children, what you can take, and what you can't.

Here are a few questions to ask yourself as you try to figure out what's best for you:

- How important is it to me to have biological children?

- If I'm married or dating someone, how does my partner feel about biological children?

- If I'm single, how do I feel about the idea of introducing frozen eggs into a future relationship? What about frozen embryos?

- What do my religious beliefs say about egg freezing or embryo freezing?

- How comfortable am I with additional medical procedures beyond my needed cancer treatments?

- How afraid am I that fertility treatment after cancer might cause my cancer to recur?

- How do I feel about the idea of undergoing fertility treatments now, before cancer treatment, and again in the future?

- How do I feel about adoption?

- What are my family members' attitudes about infertility treatments and about adoption? How important are these attitudes to me?

- How would I pay for fertility preservation or IVF? How would I pay for adoption, egg donation, or surrogacy if I choose not to pursue fertility preservation and later cannot have biological children?

- When I imagine my family ten years down the road, what does it look like?

Sample Letters of Medical Necessity for Insurers[9]

Note that the initial letter of medical necessity to your insurance carrier should come from the physician who is currently treating you, but the "appeal" letter, if your request for coverage is denied, should come from you. The most recently updated versions of both of the following sample letters can also be downloaded from the

Oncofertility Consortium's website at http://oncofertility.north western.edu/health-professionals/fertility-preservation-billing-resources.

Initial Letter to Insurer

Blue Cross Blue Shield Review Unit
By fax: (999) 999-9999
Attn: Appeals

Re:	Doe, Jane
D.O.B.:	9-30-1975
Blue Cross Blue Shield ID#:	9999999999
Group #:	99999

To Whom It May Concern:

Ms. Jane Doe is a thirty-five-year-old with stage IV colon cancer diagnosed in January 2009. The patient's plan of care for this diagnosis includes chemotherapy and likely subsequent radiation. Many of these therapies that so effectively help increase survival have side effects that may cause the loss of fertility. The patient is not currently infertile but may be rendered sterile by the cancer treatment (a benefit covered under her plan).

In preparation for these treatments, the patient saw me in consultation to review fertility preservation options as per American Society of Clinical Oncology (ASCO) and American Society for Reproductive Medicine Guidelines (attached).

After discussing the probable impact of the proposed cancer treatment on her fertility, we reviewed the range of options available.

(*Select the appropriate paragraph and delete the others.*)

After discussing the range of options available, based on her cancer treatment, age, diagnosis, and time available until the start of her cancer treatment, the decision was made to bank embryos. Embryo banking is the standard of care for fertility preservation for someone in her circumstance.

After discussing the range of options available, based on her cancer treatment, age, diagnosis, and time available until the start of her cancer treatment, the decision was made to bank eggs. Egg banking is the standard of care for fertility preservation for someone in her circumstance.

After discussing the range of options available, based on her cancer treatment, age, diagnosis, and time available until the start of her cancer treatment, the decision was made to perform a fertility sparing unilateral salpingo-oophorectomy and ovarian tissue cryopreservation prior to beginning her treatment. Surgical intervention is the standard of care for obtaining ovarian tissue for cryopreservation.

(*Note for male patients:* This can be customized to include a description of the male diagnosis. Use of sperm banking, donor sperm, and/or assisted reproductive technologies to treat couples in which the man has been rendered infertile by cancer treatment is NOT the same as infertility from other causes, and is often covered.)

Therefore, we request that this treatment as well as related procedures and testing be covered for this patient.

As noted, the patient did not present with infertility, but this fertility preservation treatment is essential to preserving fertility prior to beginning cancer treatment.

If you have any questions or need further information, please do not hesitate to contact me.

Sincerely,

John Smith, MD
Lead Physician
Center for Advanced Reproductive Services

Attachments

1. Lee, S. J., et al. 2006. American Society of Clinical Oncology recommendations on fertility preservation in cancer patients. *Journal of Clinical Oncology* 24:917–2931.

2. Ethics Committee of the American Society for Reproductive Medicine. 2005. Fertility preservation and reproduction in cancer patients. *Fertility and Sterility* 83(6):1622–28.

Sample Letter of Appeal If Initial Request for Coverage Is Denied

Blue Cross Blue Shield Review Unit
By fax: (999) 999-9999
Attn: Appeals

Re:	Doe, Jane
D.O.B.:	9-30-1975
Blue Cross Blue Shield ID#:	9999999999
Group #:	99999

To Whom It May Concern:

I am a thirty-five-year-old with stage IV colon cancer diagnosed in January 2009. My plan of care for this diagnosis includes chemotherapy and likely subsequent radiation. Many of the therapies that so effectively help increase survival have side effects that may cause the loss of fertility. I am not currently infertile but may be rendered sterile by the cancer treatment (a benefit covered under their plan).

In preparation for these treatments, I met with Dr. John Smith in consultation to review the possible impact of my cancer treatment on my fertility and my options for fertility preservation as per the American Society of Clinical Oncology (ASCO) and American Society for Reproductive Medicine Guidelines (see below).

(*Select the appropriate paragraph and delete the others.*)

After discussing the range of options available, based on my cancer treatment, age, diagnosis, and time available until the start of my cancer treatment, the decision was made to bank embryos. Embryo banking is the standard of care for fertility preservation for someone in my circumstance.

After discussing the range of options available, based on my cancer treatment, age, diagnosis, and time available until the start of my cancer treatment, the decision was made to bank eggs. Egg banking is the standard of care for fertility preservation for someone in my circumstance.

After discussing the range of options available, based on my cancer treatment, age, diagnosis, and time available until the start of my cancer treatment, the decision was made to perform a fertility sparing unilateral salpingo-oophorectomy and ovarian tissue cryopreservation prior to beginning my treatment. Surgical intervention is the standard of care for obtaining ovarian tissue for cryopreservation.

(*Note for male patients:* This can be customized to include a description of the male diagnosis if the male is the patient. Use of sperm banking, donor sperm, and/or assisted reproductive technologies to treat couples where the man has been rendered infertile by cancer treatment is NOT the same as infertility from other causes and is often covered.)

Therefore, we request that this procedure as well as related procedures and testing previously denied for coverage be reconsidered.

As noted, I do not have infertility but this treatment was essential to preserving my fertility before my cancer treatment could begin.

If you have any questions or need further information, please do not hesitate to contact me or Dr. Smith at the Center for [name of your hospital, cancer center, or fertility program].

Sincerely,

Jane Doe

Attachments

1. Lee, S. J., et al. 2006. American Society of Clinical Oncology recommendations on fertility preservation in cancer patients. *Journal of Clinical Oncology* 24:917–2931.

2. Ethics Committee of the American Society for Reproductive Medicine. 2005. Fertility preservation and reproduction in cancer patients. *Fertility and Sterility* 83(6):1622–28.

CHAPTER 3

Not So Inconceivable

Spontaneous Conception and Assisted Reproduction

WHAT IF YOU'RE UNABLE or unwilling to take on the hurdles of fertility preservation prior to treatment, and adoption just doesn't seem right for you either? What if you were diagnosed with cancer several years ago and didn't even know about the *option* of preserving your fertility? Do you still have a chance of conceiving on your own—or with a little help?

The short answer is yes. As I mentioned in chapter 1, the general rule is that the younger you were when you were treated for cancer, the better your chances are of eventually regaining your fertility, even if you got zapped with some of the nastiest chemo drugs. There are exceptions—even if you were a strapping, otherwise healthy twenty-one-year-old when you received a bone marrow transplant with full body radiation, you're pretty unlikely to get your fertility back. And if you received strong pelvic radiation as a girl, before you hit puberty, your ovarian function may never recover.

But with these few exceptions, your odds of getting your fertility back after cancer may be better than you think. As I mentioned in chapter 1, recent research has found that women under forty often have a reasonably good chance of returning to normal menstrual cycles after chemotherapy causes temporary menopause, and in one study, about a third of these women became pregnant. (It's not clear how many of them were actually *trying* to get pregnant, either.)

Just look at Lance Armstrong, who assumed that after the grueling treatment he underwent for testicular cancer in 1996, the only way he'd conceive a child would be using frozen sperm. After fathering three kids through IVF with those sperm, Armstrong and girlfriend Anna Hansen conceived son Max, born in June 2009, the old-fashioned way. "For less toxic treatments recovery often takes one to three years while for very toxic treatments (for example, preparation for a bone marrow or stem cell transplant) it may take as long as five to ten years, if normal sperm production returns at all," notes the Center for Reproductive Medicine at the Cleveland Clinic. "Recovery of sperm production after this time is rare, but it can happen."[1]

That doesn't mean you shouldn't still consider banking sperm or freezing eggs or embryos if the option is still open to you—just that you might still be able to have biological children even if the window for pursuing fertility preservation has closed.

Are You Still Fertile?

How can you tell if you're still fertile? It's more obvious for a woman than for a man. If you are no longer menstruating regularly, odds are that you are no longer fertile. (Although even this is not a 100 percent guarantee—ask the women who've had "menopause babies!") Usually, if you've gone through chemopause as a result of cancer treatment, you can expect that your menstrual cycles will return within a year of completing treatment. If it's been more than a year and they haven't come back, most doctors will say that the odds are fairly slim—although not zero—that they ever will.

But even if you're menstruating again, that doesn't mean you're fertile. It's certainly a good sign, but even women with clockwork periods may find themselves having difficulties conceiving. Just because you're having regular cycles, it doesn't mean that your ovaries are producing normal eggs that are healthy enough to conceive a pregnancy.

So assuming that your periods have come back, how can you tell if you're likely to be fertile? One option is to seek out the advice of a fertility specialist, usually called a *reproductive endocrinologist*. You can find a doctor who is a member of the American Society of Reproductive Medicine on their website at https://www.asrm.org/euclid/detail.aspx?id=2328.

One of the first tests a fertility specialist will do measures something called your day 3 *follicle-stimulating hormone* (FSH). An FSH test measures how much of this hormone your body is producing in the effort to coax an egg to mature and release. If your ovaries are running low on eggs, your body senses this and produces more FSH as it tries to stimulate the ovaries to produce a good egg. There's no absolute "you can't get pregnant now!" cut-off for FSH levels, but the lower they are, the better. Most specialists in cancer and fertility like to see FSH levels at 10 or below. The higher your FSH levels are, the more likely it is that you'll need assistance getting pregnant.

Most insurance companies do at least cover initial fertility consultation and testing, such as blood work, even if they don't actually pay for fertility treatments. Others don't—although, just as with egg and embryo freezing before cancer treatment, you may be able to persuade your insurance company to cover fertility services for you because your infertility is likely a "side effect of a covered treatment." Simply modify the sample letters from chapter 2 to describe your situation (or have your doctor's office do so).

If you can't get coverage, or if you're anxious about going in for an office visit when you're not sure if you really have a problem, you can also take an at-home fertility test from First Response, which makes pregnancy and ovulation tests. These tests cost between $15 and $25 and are available from pretty much any drugstore—sometimes coming in packs of two or four. Instead of having the fertility specialist take your blood on day three of your menstrual cycle, you pee on a stick on that day. The test has its limits—it doesn't tell you your exact FSH level but just says if you're "fertile" or "not fertile." If the test line that shows up in the little window is darker than the "reference line," then you're likely to have elevated FSH levels and should move ahead with scheduling that appointment at the fertility clinic. If it's lighter than the reference line, or if no test line shows up at all, then you might consider trying to conceive "unassisted" for a few months.

Obviously, you'll get a lot more detailed testing and information from a visit to a fertility specialist. But if you want to check things out in the privacy of your own home first, this is an inexpensive way to do it. Just remember that a "good" result—low FSH levels—is not an absolute promise that you're still fertile, because FSH is only one way to assess your fertility.

Men who want to test their sperm motility at home used to be able to use a dual version of the at-home fertility test, called Fertell. Unfortunately, it doesn't seem to be on the market in the United States anymore. Most places that used to sell it now say that it's out of stock, so sperm testing is pretty much reserved for your doctor's office for now.

When Should You Get Pregnant?

Whether you want to try getting pregnant on your own or you're seeking fertility treatments, as a cancer survivor you have some timing issues to think about.

Most of these questions primarily affect women. For a guy, the whole question of when to try for children is a lot easier. Since you make new sperm constantly, there's really not a lot of concern about "damaged" sperm in your ejaculate after cancer treatment. Once you're a month or two out from treatment, it's unlikely that there's anything wrong with the new swimmers in your semen. And although the first two years after treatment are your time of greatest risk for the cancer's returning, you're not going to be the one who's pregnant—so if it does, you won't have to choose between starting treatment right away and taking a pregnancy to term.

For women, first there's the worry about how much, and if, your cancer treatments may have damaged your eggs. That is, what if the egg you conceive with has chromosomal damage from the chemotherapy drugs you've taken? It's true that many chemo drugs can, in fact, wreak havoc on the DNA of a woman's developing eggs.

There is no research that indicates that women who have undergone chemotherapy have a long-term risk of having a baby with chromosomal abnormalities. But most experts in the field agree that it is best to wait six months to a year after completing chemotherapy before attempting to get pregnant. "That seems to be a sufficiently long period to allow any damaged eggs to clear your system," says Dr. Oktay. Eggs that have been significantly damaged by chemotherapy usually do not survive within a woman's reproductive system any longer than that.

There's another reason to wait a bit after completing cancer treatment of any kind before you try to conceive: the risk of recurrence. Pregnancy itself doesn't appear to increase the risk of your cancer's returning (more on that in chapter 6), but most doctors will tell you that cancer survivors are at the greatest risk of having their disease come back during the first two years after treatment—especially if the cancer is one of the more aggressive ones. (Women with hormone-positive breast cancer appear to have a longer window of time during which their risk of recurrence remains relatively high.) If you do become pregnant during this time, and then your disease returns, you have some very difficult decisions to make.

Christina Demosthenous was in a position like this. It wasn't a recurrence, but her first breast cancer diagnosis. She was thirty-two, and the lump she felt in her breast seemed like nothing. Then, when she got pregnant, her breasts began to change and the lump seemed to disappear. But her obstetrician urged her to get further tests. "Pregnancy and cancer don't mix," he said.

Christina was three months pregnant when she was finally diagnosed with breast cancer—a type that was highly sensitive to hormone levels. "I live in New York and I went to see about every doctor in town," she says. "Nobody said, 'Don't worry about it, just have surgery and chemo and it will all be okay.' They all just said, 'Ugh, this is bad.' Two doctors finally looked at me and advised me to terminate the pregnancy. I didn't care if I died, I wanted this baby more than anything else in the world, but I thought to myself, if it doesn't turn out good, I would be even more devastated to think I wouldn't be around for my baby." Ending her pregnancy, Christina says, was the hardest decision she ever had to make.

Some women may be able to sustain a pregnancy after being diagnosed with cancer—especially if the cancer diagnosis or recurrence comes late in the pregnancy, when you're closer to the time when an early C-section and immediate treatment might be feasible. Although Carly Chandler, who later adopted from foster care, also found a lump in her breast early on in her second pregnancy, it wasn't diagnosed as cancer until much later, when she was able to deliver her son early and begin treatment.

Christina actually might have gotten different advice about her original pregnancy if she'd been diagnosed more recently. A new study that came out in 2009 indicates that if the worst happens and you *do* get diagnosed with breast cancer, or a recurrence, while pregnant, you might not have to end the pregnancy. Researchers at MD Anderson Cancer Center found that there was no difference in the odds of surviving ten years between the women who were not pregnant during or slightly before their diagnosis, and those who were. You shouldn't start chemotherapy during your first trimester, the researchers said, but when chemo begins in the second or third trimester, babies are just as healthy as those born to mothers without breast cancer.[2]

Still, you really don't want to risk being put in that position if you don't have to. So most experts say it's best to wait at least two years after completing cancer treatment before becoming pregnant.

On the other hand, as mentioned previously, you don't want to wait *too* long. As a cancer survivor, especially if you've undergone chemotherapy, the odds are that you will go into menopause earlier than you otherwise would have. So even if your cycles have come back, and you're fertile now, you may not stay that way as long as you might expect. "In all likelihood, this will shorten your fertile years," says Dr. Lee.

So you have to strike a balance: take the time to finish treatment and have a couple of "safe" recurrence-free years, but time your efforts so that you're not just starting to try to conceive at thirty-eight when you might hit early menopause at forty. If you're thirty-five, two years out of treatment and know you want a child, but it's not the right time—your husband's deploying, you're changing careers, whatever—you might want to consider freezing eggs or embryos *now*, just in case.

And for a few women, it may be advisable to try to get pregnant sooner than that two-year window. Some young women with early-stage, low-grade endometrial cancers choose to take a conservative approach to treatment—hormonal treatment that leaves their uterus intact—because they do want to bear children and don't want an immediate hysterectomy. If your doctor agrees with this treatment plan, you might want to start your family sooner rather than later, so that you can then have more definitive surgical treatment as soon as you're finished having children.

Getting Pregnant on Your Own

You might be surprised at just how many cancer survivors have gotten pregnant on their own, with no help from technology at all.

Christina Demosthenous was so eager to try again to have a baby, after her heartbreaking experience being diagnosed with cancer in early pregnancy, that she literally kept a calendar counting the days until she and her husband could begin their quest again. Her doctor agreed that she could take a break from Tamoxifen after two years on the drug, and the two-year mark was circled on her calendar in red.

"Then when I went to my oncologist, she said, 'I told you *that*?'" Christina recalls. Her doctor tried to persuade her to stay on the medication longer, citing its powerful benefits in women who are hormone receptor positive, but Christina was adamant. "I said, I really want to have a baby and I want to have it now."

She went off Tamoxifen, and waited the three months that doctors advised to let the medication clear out of her system. "I got pregnant the first month we started trying!" she marvels. "We swore it would take forever, but it happened right away. I think we just got the timing right." In January 2009, she gave birth to her son Plato.

As soon as Christina gave birth, her oncologist handed her a new Tamoxifen prescription. "I couldn't fill it. I knew I would want another child and I wouldn't want to wait five years. And it's not like you can start up and stop again six months later," she says. "So we're trying again now. This time, it's not happening as quickly, but as soon as this baby is born, I'll go back on Tamoxifen." So far, she has remained hopeful and cancer-free.

Kristine Schmalenberg, who adopted a son in Kazakhstan, initially elected not to interrupt her Tamoxifen to try to get pregnant. But as she neared the four-year mark, she decided to take the leap. "I went off the drug at four years, without talking to my oncologist," she confesses. "I didn't want her to tell me no!" Like Christina Demosthenous, she waited a few months for the drug to leave her system, then started trying to conceive. At thirty-six, four years after undergoing chemotherapy known to be toxic to fertility, it took her just three months to become pregnant. "We weren't really optimistic and were prepared for it to take a lot longer, so we were thrilled when it happened so soon!" she says. Today, older son Max is five and little brother Bennett is three.

Even Lindsay Nohr Beck, who froze eggs before chemotherapy for tongue cancer, then used IVF with preimplantation genetic diagnosis to get pregnant with her daughter after learning of the genetic abnormality that her husband could pass along, ended up having her second child without any assistance at all.

"We had gone through a couple of IVF cycles to try to get pregnant again, and I miscarried," she says. "So we decided to take the summer off from the IVF roller coaster, and I got pregnant accidentally." She thought she'd miscarry again—her husband's balanced translocation had led to a series of miscarriages before they discovered the problem. "At every appointment, I'd expect that there would be no sac or no heartbeat, that we'd have a tough decision to make. But at each test, the news was great. Our son Walker is one in a million."

Of course, Lindsay was twenty-nine when she had her daughter through IVF, and in her early thirties when she had Walker. But even if you're old enough to remember the Carter administration, that doesn't necessarily mean there's no hope at all of getting pregnant.

I was forty when my husband and I decided to start trying to conceive. We had adopted our beautiful daughter less than two years earlier, but the agency we had used for her adoption was reputed to be having some problems. (They later shut down.) We were nervous about working with them again and at the same time daunted by the prospect of researching more agencies and trying to find one we could trust. Then I said to my husband, "You know, no one ever told us I *couldn't* get pregnant. We just assumed I wouldn't be able to."

By then, I was more than two years past my initial treatment, and the cancer hadn't reared its ugly head. We hadn't been actively trying to prevent a pregnancy, but we hadn't been taking a very systematic approach to conceive one, either. So we decided that, while we researched new agencies, we might as well try *really really hard* to get pregnant. For us, that meant first taking a home fertility test to reassure me that it was worth getting all excited about. I took the only test then on the market, Fertell, fully expecting it to not only show that I had fertility problems, but to actually sit up on the back of the toilet tank and point and laugh at me. I was forty years old and a cancer survivor, after all.

It didn't. It said things were clear for takeoff. In our next nod to technology, we bought the Clearblue Easy Fertility Monitor— the fancy schmancy digital doodad that takes readings of your first morning's pee and tells you not only when you're about to ovulate, but alerts you on the days when you're *getting ready* to ovulate, days when you're also increasingly fertile and should make plenty of time for "baby dancing."

The first month we used it, the Clearblue Monitor started telling me I was in my "high" fertility phase at about day ten of my cycle. We dutifully began hitting the sheets at every opportunity. I kept waiting for the little test window to show a tiny digital egg, the sign that I was about to ovulate—but it never did. From cycle day ten to cycle day twenty-four or so, I just kept getting high readings. We were getting a bit tired, but we kept up our marathon. Eventually, the reading just dropped back down to low again, and I figured I either hadn't ovulated that month, or the machine just didn't "get" me yet. (It's supposed to learn the fluctuations of your menstrual cycle the longer you use it.)

Dejected, we thought we'd try again next month. But we didn't have to. A day or so before my next period was due, I couldn't resist taking a home pregnancy test. A few minutes later, I stumbled out of the bathroom in the predawn light, waving the stick in Evan's face, yelping "Is that a line? I think it's a line!!" It was . . . and nine mostly uneventful months later, six weeks before I turned forty-one, that line turned into our beautiful, six-pound, three-ounce son Adrian.

When Adrian was about eighteen months old, and his big sister three, we decided that maybe we weren't quite done yet. That time, it took two months of trying (and the help of the good old Clearblue Easy Fertility monitor again) for me to get pregnant with our daughter, Katia. I was forty-three when she was born on June 17, 2010—seven pounds, ten ounces of gorgeous perfection.

To be fair, not everyone's postcancer pregnancy goes entirely smoothly—although the outcomes can be just as joyful. Terri Turner had adopted a daughter from Colombia in 2007, six years after being diagnosed with breast cancer at the age of twenty-nine. She and her husband were in the process of filling out the paperwork to adopt again when they decide to try to get pregnant on their own. Terri was worried about recurrence, but she knew her husband really wanted to try for a biological child.

"I was scared out of my mind, not trusting my body. As it turned out, it was the world's most harrowing pregnancy, like an eight-month plane crash," she says. "The whole time, I was thinking, why the bleep did I not adopt again? It turned out that my son had a lump on the umbilical cord that was constricting blood flow, so the poor little guy was just starving for eight months. I'd do kick counts constantly and if I didn't feel him, I'd rush in, thinking he was dying. They don't know why it happened. I made it to thirty-six weeks and a scheduled C-section, and Nikolai was born at three pounds, five ounces. He was a tiny, scary-skinny little chicken. Now he's big and beautiful and fabulous."

Seeking Fertility Assistance

In some cases, cancer survivors might want to use assisted reproduction to become pregnant even if they aren't necessarily having any fertility problems. For example, doctors may recommend that young women who've had conservative treatment (hormones only, no hysterectomy) for early-stage endometrial cancer consider using IVF to help them become pregnant as soon as possible. That way, they can complete their family more quickly and undergo a hysterectomy, which offers more definitive protection against the return of endometrial cancer.

And while most cancers are *not* inherited, some are. For example, if you have a BRCA1 or BRCA2 genetic mutation, which confers a drastically heightened risk for breast cancer and ovarian cancer, you have a fifty-fifty chance of passing it on to your daughters. For that reason, some women with these mutations choose to plan their families using IVF with preimplantation genetic diagnosis (PGD). This means that during the IVF process, one cell is removed from each fertilized embryo and tested for the BRCA mutation. That way, only embryos that don't carry the cancer-causing mutation can be implanted. When you've seen sisters, mothers, aunts, and cousins face breast cancer and perhaps die from it, it's understandable to want to spare your daughters the same fate.

Or you simply may not have had the opportunity to try to preserve eggs, embryos, or sperm prior to cancer treatment. Maybe your doctor didn't mention it to you, or maybe it was all just too overwhelming at the time. But now, two years or five years or ten years down the road, you're hoping that there might still be a chance that you're fertile, and you want to try to become pregnant or father a child.

It could be possible. Men have pretty much no way of knowing if there is functional semen in their sperm without testing, but for women there are more signs. If you stopped having menstrual periods entirely after your cancer treatment, and they never came back, the odds are slim. But as long as you're not in total menopause, with no ovarian function left at all, it's entirely possible that you might still have some eggs left. You may not be able to get pregnant on your own, but with the help of fertility treatments, it could be a possibility. Similarly, men who are unsure of whether or not they still might be fertile after cancer treatment should consult a fertility specialist. You could be like Lance Armstrong and father a child spontaneously more than a decade after you thought your sperm were wiped out!

If you're able to, your best bet for fertility treatments that take into account your unique circumstances as a cancer survivor is to go to a fertility program that is in some way affiliated with a cancer center (part of the same medical center, for example) or has an oncofertility specialty. You can find a program like this through organizations like Fertile Hope/Livestrong and the Oncofertil-ity Consortium (see Resources). Staff at such programs will be a lot more knowledgeable about issues such as whether or not specific fertility medications—in particular, those that raise the estrogen levels in your body—might raise your risk of recurrence, and what other options you might have. Look back at chapter 2 for further information about some of the fertility treatments you might undergo at one of these programs.

If getting pregnant on your own still isn't an option, there are other avenues to consider. Some cancer survivors have success-fully built their families using egg donors or surrogates, and you'll read more about those options in the next chapter.

CHAPTER 4

Third-Party Lines

Embryo or Egg Donation and Surrogacy

WHAT IF YOUR CANCER TREATMENT has left you definitely unable to conceive or carry your own pregnancy, but you're uncomfortable with traditional adoption—or at least, you'd like to explore other options?

There are a couple of other possibilities. If conceiving the pregnancy is your primary issue—if your ovaries no longer function—then you could consider donor eggs or embryos. If it's your uterus that is the problem, then you could look into having a surrogate carry a pregnancy for you.

Egg and Embryo Donation

As you know, many women who've survived cancer discover that their ovaries no longer work the way they once did. They may be in early menopause, or they may get their menstrual cycles back but still find themselves unable to conceive a pregnancy. But that doesn't mean they couldn't *carry* a pregnancy to term and have a healthy baby—just that they can't get one started in the first place.

Remember, the uterus ages much more slowly than the ovaries do, and even women in menopause can safely and healthily carry a pregnancy to term once the embryo is securely implanted in the uterus. For families in this situation, egg and embryo donation are two options to consider.

If your male partner has no trouble with his sperm, you have the option of egg donation. "The biggest category of people using donated eggs are people who've gone through premature ovarian failure," says Marybeth Gerrity of the Oncofertility Consortium. "That includes a lot of people who've gone through cancer, such as those who didn't get counseling about fertility preservation before treatment. If your uterus is still intact and undamaged, it gives you the opportunity to experience pregnancy, and the baby can at least be genetically related to your husband."

For most egg donors, says Gerrity, a cancer history isn't an issue. "It may not even be much noted in your file that infertility related to cancer is your reason for pursuing egg donation, especially for people who've had childhood cancers."

If you type "egg donation" into a search engine, you'll find dozens of agencies that offer this service, allowing you to choose from egg donors by age, race, appearance, academic profile, and a number of other factors. (To be honest, some of these sites look more like modeling portfolios than assisted reproduction programs!) These women are compensated for donating eggs—usually between $5,000 and $10,000, but it's not unfair to say that a five-foot, seven-inch, 125-pound, blonde, blue-eyed star athlete who graduated from Harvard could probably command a bit more. Gerrity recommends staying away from the "vanity" programs and, instead, searching for an egg donation program that is affiliated with a respected infertility center. You can find them, and search their success rates, through the Society for Assisted Reproductive Technology and their website at www.sart.org.

The egg donation process generally works this way:

1. You sign up with an agency or program and choose a donor. If she's available, a short profile of your family will be presented to her.

2. Once a donor agrees to match with you, often both you and the donor will go through psychological testing. Your agency will then walk you through the process of signing a legal contract. Both you and your donor should have legal representation. (Guess what—you usually pay for both.)

3. Once you've finalized an agreement—usually requiring a substantial up-front deposit, if not the entire fee in advance—the intended mother and the egg donor go through a process of medical treatment to synchronize cycles. The egg donor's side of the process is pretty much exactly like standard IVF, except that instead of retrieving eggs to be fertilized and implanted in her own uterus (or frozen for later implantation), the eggs are instead fertilized with sperm from the recipient father and then implanted in the intended mother's uterus. The process is a lot simpler for the intended mom—basically, you would take a course of medication designed to prepare the lining of your uterus for implantation of embryos.

4. Between two and four embryos are implanted. Any remaining embryos are usually frozen for later use.

5. You wait to see if you're pregnant!

So what does all this cost? It varies—of course. But it's not cheap. The Egg Donor Program, a California-based agency, indicates on their website that they charge between $6,000 and $7,500 for their services (including matching, psychological evaluations, legal representation for both parties, and coordinating the IVF cycle). Donors receive between $7,000 and $8,000 for the first cycle. And then there are the medical expenses for the actual egg retrieval, implantation and storage—which, as you learned in previous chapters, can run between $15,000 and $20,000. So you can assume that the whole process is probably going to cost at least $30,000.

Is any of it paid for by insurance? You might be surprised. "Here in Illinois, donor egg insemination is covered by insurance, if you've lost ovarian function because of cancer treatment or surgical removal of the ovaries to treat a medical condition. It's not unusual for an insurance policy that covers IVF to cover egg donation," says Gerrity. Even the donor fee? "Usually, yes, they do cover the fee to the donor up to a 'usual and customary' range. They may not pay the $30,000 to get an egg from some 'premiere' agency, but that's not what most donors are getting anyway."

Illinois is one of the states with generally better insurance coverage for assisted reproductive technology, so that might not be the case in *your* state—but here, as with IVF and fertility preservation, you might be able to get your insurer to make an exception. "Some states don't cover anything," Gerrity says. "But you can use the same sample letters we provide to request case-by-case coverage for fertility preservation and IVF for egg donation; just modify the letter to reflect your course of treatment. And be sure to mention that your infertility is a known side effect of a covered treatment, *not* a result of voluntary sterilization, and that egg donation is a standard and accepted form of care for your condition. Donor sperm is often covered for men; certainly, the insurance company wouldn't want to be perceived as covering treatment for one sex and not the other!"

You can also get pregnant using embryo donation. Today, according to RESOLVE, the national infertility organization, there are more than 400,000 cryopreserved embryos sitting in storage around the country. Most of them, of course, are intended to be used by the couple who conceived them. And honestly, says Gerrity, embryo donation will probably never become a common practice. "In general, fertility patients aren't excited about donating embryos," she says. "Once they've completed their family and have embryos in storage, they're more likely to consider a donation to research. The idea of somebody out there raising their child is not something they're excited about."

But it certainly does happen. There are a number of agencies and organizations that arrange embryo adoptions today, including the well-known Nightlight Christian Adoptions and the National Embryo Donation Center. Some fertility centers themselves also offer embryo donation programs.

Kim Walton is among several families who founded Miracles Waiting (www.miracleswaiting.org), a nonprofit information and support organization focused on embryo adoption. Members (it's free to join) can find listings of both prospective embryo donors and prospective adoptive families. Not surprisingly, there are more prospective families on the site than donors, but the number of donors has been climbing. "During 2009, we got about seven donor members for every ten recipient members, so there's not that much of a disparity," Walton says. "In some months, we truly saw parity, and we're getting close to the same number of donors as recipients. The word is getting out that there is this other alternative."

Walton says that, as far as she knows, they haven't had any families with a cancer history adopt embryos through Miracles Waiting, but that it certainly wouldn't rule people out of embryo adoption. "I think this is a great avenue for someone with a cancer history who wants to carry their own child, experience pregnancy, and control how the baby is cared for in utero, but who can't conceive using their own eggs," she says.

Agency-arranged embryo adoptions generally require a home study, just as with "standard" adoptions, but independent embryo adoptions may not. "Miracles Waiting doesn't require it, but certainly allows for it," says Walton. "It's truly up to the donor family. I would say fewer ask for it than do not ask for it, but it is a concern to some people."

Embryo adoption may be less costly than egg donation. Walton estimates that most embryo adoptions arranged with the assistance of Miracles Waiting cost a total of $4,000 to $5,000, depending on what the clinic charges. As with egg donation, you may be able to get some or all of these costs covered by an insurance company if you approach them in the right way (use the Oncofertility Consortium sample letters and adapt them to your specific situation).

Surrogacy

If you're still fertile, but you can't carry a pregnancy to term—for example, if your uterus has been damaged by radiation—you might still be able to have a biological child if that's very important to you. You can use IVF techniques to fertilize one of your eggs with your partner's sperm, and then have a gestational surrogate carry the baby. Actually, even if you're *not* still fertile, you could use your partner's sperm to fertilize a donor egg and then have an unrelated surrogate carry the pregnancy to term. Or if you have eggs or embryos frozen from before you began treatment, you can engage a surrogate to carry them.

"The most common reason cancer survivors use a gestational carrier is because they've lost their uterus, or it has been so badly damaged by radiation that it can't sustain a pregnancy," says Gerrity. "For some breast cancer patients, their doctors are still concerned about the high estrogen levels of pregnancy and the risk of cancer recurrence." Ovaries are also removed in some women with early-stage hormone-positive breast cancer to induce menopause.

You can find a surrogate in one of two ways. First, there are surrogacy programs—some independent and some affiliated with major medical centers, like the one at Yale University. Second, you can find the surrogate yourself, either through networking among friends, relatives, and acquaintances, or by making connections through surrogacy networks such as surromomsonline.com.

Many families have successfully found surrogates without using a center. Gerrity, however, recommends the protection of an established program. "There are always ways you can get stuff cheaper off the Internet; sometimes it works, sometimes it doesn't. There's not a review system where people are rating the last vendor, and sometimes there will be scam artists," she says. "The best way to pursue surrogacy is to go to a reliable IVF center that does a lot of third-party reproduction."

One of the reasons for this is that surrogacy laws vary widely from state to state—even more so than with adoption. In fact, in some states, surrogacy contracts are not recognized as legally binding at all, so if something disrupts the process, the parents who've engaged the surrogate may have no legal recourse. "Every state is a little different about whose baby this is legally, not just biologically," Gerrity says. "In some states, even when you use donor eggs, the baby carried by the surrogate is automatically your baby. In other states, you'll have to legally adopt that baby. Be very careful that you know what the regulations are in the state where you're receiving your treatment. And think beyond just the financial aspects. Be sure that person carrying a pregnancy for you will give you the baby at the end. Make sure you know the behaviors that person is going to be engaging in during the pregnancy." Whether or not you work with a surrogacy program or center or independently, you and your surrogate will both need an attorney to draw up your contract and represent your interests.

After a recurrence of Michelle Whitlock's cervical cancer forced her to have a radical hysterectomy, she elected to try to find a surrogate on her own—a process that was ultimately long and arduous. "First, I talked to a friend whom I hadn't seen in years. She had heard what was going on with me, and she had been considering becoming a surrogate but didn't know how to get into it," Michelle says. "I began researching the laws about surrogacy in her state, but she then had something go wrong with her marriage and told me she couldn't do it. So my first hopes were dashed."

Michelle began telling anyone who would listen that she was looking for a surrogate. "At a homeowner's association meeting, a woman from the management company told me she had a friend who'd always wanted to be a surrogate," she says. "It took me about four weeks to convince myself to call and talk to this stranger, but when I finally did, she said, 'Oh, I was hoping you'd call!' We met for lunch and it was kind of like 'girlfriend love at first sight.' She wasn't doing it so much for the money—she just loved being pregnant, but she didn't want any more children. So she was willing to do it for $5,000."

Michelle and the surrogate, Trista, worked out a contract (which included a psychological evaluation), and in September 2008, they thawed and implanted three frozen embryos that Michelle had preserved prior to her initial treatment. "We got a positive pregnancy test and were over the moon excited," she says. "Then we went in for the first ultrasound and they told us it was a blighted ovum. It was terrible. Trista was emotionally overwhelmed, and she just couldn't do it again."

So Michelle went to surromomsonline.com, one of a number of online matching services for surrogate mothers and hopeful parents (some also match parents with egg and sperm donors). "I started emailing anyone within a four-hour drive," she says. She ended up meeting with another prospective surrogate, Janelle, and her family, and something just felt right. "I've worked in retail for seventeen years, and I've hired a lot of people, and I just got a good feeling." Janelle requested a fee of $15,000, plus a food allowance and medical costs not covered by her insurance.

In February 2009, Michelle had three embryos thawed. Two were implanted in Janelle's womb, and one took. "I was ecstatic, but at the same time I kind of held back. I needed to see an ultrasound with a heartbeat. When we got that, I ran out of the ultrasound room yelling, 'We've got a baby, we've got a baby!' and the clinic just kind of went crazy with me."

During her pregnancy, Janelle, a married nursing student, would come and stay with Michelle for weekends, sometimes accompanied by her youngest child. Or Michelle would visit for Janelle's doctor's appointments. "It was pretty cool—under normal circumstances, our lives wouldn't have crossed, but I think that we're blessed to have a friend we would have never met who will be part of our lives forever," Michelle says.

On October 27, Michelle and her husband were both in the delivery room with Janelle as her mom coached her through the birth of seven-pound, thirteen-ounce Riley Grier. "The three of us and the baby stayed in the hospital for forty-eight hours together," says Michelle. "Janelle's been pumping milk for us and sends us chests full of it. I've been up to visit her because her dad had cancer and she was going through a rough time. It's an amazing thing."

Michelle believes the whole journey was worth it. "She's so beautiful. I can even look back and say that I don't think my cancer was such a bad thing after all. Had I not had that cancer, I wouldn't have frozen that egg and that sperm. Although I might have a child, I wouldn't have *this* child. I feel like it all worked out the way it was supposed to," she says.

Amanda Twinam was twenty-eight and in the process of going through fertility treatments when she was diagnosed with breast cancer in August 2007. "The gynecologist found the lump during a routine exam, when I'd already gone through a cycle and a half of intrauterine insemination," she says.

The day after her mastectomy, in October, while still in the hospital, Amanda started the injections to prepare her body for the process of harvesting eggs to freeze as embryos. "I had already done all the research and had a relationship with a reproductive endocrinologist, so I was very fortunate to have all that help lined up," she says. "Honestly, I don't know if I would have done it after the cancer diagnosis had it not already been in the works. It was so overwhelming. We met with the doctor, and I walked out thinking, 'I don't know if I can do this on top of everything else.'"

Interrupting the fertility process to cope with cancer was awful, Amanda says. "Honestly, that was my big focus, much more than the cancer. I had already spent fourteen months trying to have a baby, and I had some other health issues related to fertility so I knew I would probably be high risk even if I did get pregnant. And now this?"

After chemotherapy, Amanda began taking Tamoxifen. But due to an unusual neurological reaction, her doctors stopped that drug and put her on aromatase inhibitors instead—drugs that are only for postmenopausal women, so her ovarian function was also suppressed. "Between my history of unexplained infertility, my other health problems, and my need to stay on hormonal treatments, the thought of using our embryos myself made me nervous," she says. "I was at a much higher risk of miscarriage, and we just had those nine embryos. I couldn't make any more."

So she began looking into surrogacy. In New York, where the Twinams live, surrogacy is not recognized and contracts are not enforceable. "I have a lot of friends who have offered to do it for me, but it's hard to do here, and because it's not recognized, you have to go through a whole adoption proceeding," Amanda says. "I'm a lawyer, so it makes me nervous to do it in a place where the law is like that. I know too much about what can go wrong."

So Amanda and her husband settled on a surrogacy agency in New Jersey that she'd read about in a *New York Times* magazine feature. "The woman who runs the agency is an attorney who's had three children via surrogacy herself, and has essentially 'made' the law in this area. She's a very well-respected practitioner in the field, and that's important to me because I'm a paranoid lawyer!"

In the early spring of 2010, the Twinams submitted their application to the surrogacy agency—Amanda's cancer history was never an issue—and waited for a match to be made. "They also get a thirteen-page, in-depth application from the surrogate, and if the agency thinks we're a potential match, they give us the profile," Amanda explains. "Then we have a week to decide if we want to schedule a phone conference with the surrogate to see if we're all interested in moving forward."

In late summer 2010, the Twinams were officially matched with a surrogate and were eager to begin the next steps to becoming parents. Amanda compares the lack of control she's felt during the process to the experience of cancer treatment. "You know, that lost feeling where you're being swept along by outside forces and there are no guarantees of a happy outcome. You just keep doing what you're supposed to be doing, but the stress and uncertainty can be wearing," she acknowledges. "It's a long road, and I feel like we're still at the starting gate. Some of it has been our specific requirements. I wanted a surrogate in a state where we can get a prebirth order, putting us on the birth certificate before the birth even occurs. Also, the agency is getting a lot of surrogates now who don't have their own health insurance, and the only policy you can get that includes surrogacy is $30,000—which we don't have! So we needed someone who has her own insurance."

Indeed, surrogacy isn't cheap. In fact, of all the paths to parenthood in this book, it's probably fair to say that using a surrogate is the most costly. Most surrogacy agencies estimate costs ranging from $70,000 to upwards of $100,000. Whitlock calculates that, all told, it cost her about $100,000 to have Riley—that includes compensation and medical costs and other expenses for both Janelle and Trista, as well as attorney fees, psychological testing, and other costs. She'd saved year-end bonuses for years, as well as fees she'd received for public speaking on cervical cancer and the HPV test. "I knew for five years this was the only way for us to have a baby, so when we got any extra money, it went to this," she says. "But I was still a little short and had to take out a $10,000 loan."

Amanda Twinam estimates that the surrogacy process will ultimately cost them between $70,000 and $90,000. "Some of it we're taking out of savings. I was pretty sick on chemo and never left the house, so I pretty much saved my entire paycheck—and my job was awesome. They kept paying me even when I didn't deserve it," she says. "We also sold our house. We'd built this big beautiful colonial in a good school district, with a short commute, where we'd live and raise our kids. But after I was sick, the house didn't make a lot of sense for us at that point, and the cost was pretty high. So we sold it and moved into something much smaller, and set a big chunk of that money aside."

Many health insurance companies are also now putting *surrogacy exclusions* in place for maternity care. Apparently, they don't care for the idea of covering a pregnancy that is really for the "benefit" of someone other than the person they've insured and for which the surrogate is also getting compensation. Of course, it's always possible not to tell the insurance company how the surrogate got pregnant, but you're taking the risk that they will figure it out and drop her from coverage either now or later, or even prosecute for insurance fraud. (Remember, her insurance company will be expecting her to be submitting claims for pediatrician visits and so forth, something she's not going to be doing.) And there's virtually no chance that *your* insurance company will pay for the maternity care of your surrogate, someone who's not insured under your plan.

Don't assume that your surrogate's health plan covers surrogate pregnancy, and don't try to fool them. Instead, you or your surrogate should contact her insurer before you get started and confirm that they will cover surrogate pregnancy. If they say yes, get it in writing. If they say no, you'll probably need to pay the premiums on a backup plan that *does* cover surrogate pregnancy, which can be costly, as the Twinams found out.

"Surrogacy *is* a business," says Amanda." It's hard to be the person on this side of it because it's so emotional, as the intended parent. But you don't want to be the 'difficult one' when people have your future in their hands."

If egg donation or surrogacy isn't for you, one of the most popular and successful paths to parenthood for cancer survivors is the same one undertaken by many families who've never faced cancer: adoption. You might think that cancer survivors would have trouble adopting, but although they may face a few more hurdles than the average family, the adoption process may be easier than you think. Read on!

CHAPTER 5

Be My Baby

Adoption

"WHY DON'T YOU JUST ADOPT?"

A lot of people pursuing fertility treatments get that question, and people who are worried about whether they can have children after cancer treatment are no exception. And it's a good question—except for the "just" part. Whether or not you're a cancer survivor, you don't "just" adopt. It's not a simple solution, any more than fertility treatments are simple.

But it's also not out of your reach if you're a cancer survivor, contrary to what a lot of people think. You may fear that agencies will turn you away or that a pregnant woman considering placing her child for adoption will never pick you or that you won't even pass a home study. In most cases, you'd be wrong. Nobody keeps any statistics on this, but just based on conversations with agencies and cancer survivors, and reading posts to cancer websites and adoption mailing lists, I'd venture to bet that hundreds, if not thousands, of cancer survivors have been able to adopt children. You could be one of them—if it's right for you.

How Does Adoption Work?

This is a book about having children after cancer, not about adoption itself, so I'm not going to delve too far into the fine details of the adoption process. There are other books designed to do just that, and you can find a list of some of them in the Resources section at the end of this book. Still, when you're thinking about whether or not you can, should, and want to adopt as a cancer survivor, it's important to know the basics.

There are three general ways to adopt in the United States: *private domestic adoption, international adoption*, and *foster-adoption*. When I say "private domestic adoption," I'm talking about any and all adoptions of a child from the United States, in which the state has *not* already taken temporary or permanent custody of the child away from the birth parents. That can mean adopting through an agency or using an attorney. (Four states—Colorado, Connecticut, Delaware, and Massachusetts—require you to use an agency for adoptions and do not permit attorney-managed adoptions.)

Domestic adoptions can be *open* (birth parents have direct contact with the adoptive family through letters, emails, phone calls, and often even visits); *semi-open* (birth parents have more limited contact with the adoptive family, sometimes only through an intermediary like an agency or attorney); or *closed* (neither the birth family nor the adoptive family has any information about each other, and there is no contact). The trend in domestic adoption has been away from fully closed adoptions, since many professionals now believe that, in most cases, at least some degree of openness is good for everyone involved.

International adoption means just what it says: adopting a child from another country. For virtually all international adoptions to the United States, you have to go through an accredited agency. Most international adoptions used to be closed, since it was often difficult to locate the birth parents of a child adopted from another country, but that has changed in recent years. Many parents adopting children internationally strive to maintain some kind of relationship with their child's birth family, if they are known and can be located.

Adoption from foster care means that the child (or children) you are adopting has been taken from the birth parents' custody by some state authority—usually your state's version of a family services agency. With foster-adoption, the child is sometimes placed in your care as a foster child while the state is still considering whether or not the birth parents can eventually parent him or her again. Sometimes, on the other hand, foster children are already free for adoption because their birth parents' rights have already been severed. Usually, these are older children.

Cancer survivors can, and have, adopted children using all of these options. Which is right for you? It depends on a lot of factors, some having to do with your cancer diagnosis and some that you'd have to consider whether or not you were a cancer survivor.

Questions to Ask When Choosing an Adoption Path

Answering the questions below can help you to further define your expectations and pinpoint what type of adoption might be right for you and your family.

- What do I picture my future child and family looking like? How attached am I to that specific picture?

- Is it very important to me (and my partner, if I have one) to parent a newborn or very young baby?

- How do I/we feel about openness in adoption? What degree of openness am I comfortable with?

- What are my extended family's attitudes about adoption? If they're negative, how would I educate them? If they don't take well to the information I give them, what would I do then?

- Would I be comfortable parenting a child of another race or ethnicity? Do I have the resources, and am I willing to spend the time, to make sure my child is connected to his or her race or heritage?

- Can I take time off from work to travel to, and spend time in, another country to visit and bring my child home? (Korea is about the only country that does not require at least one overseas trip by adoptive parents; some require two or more.)

- How hard would it be for me to parent a baby or child for several months, then have to return the child to his birth parents if the foster care plan called for reunification?

- What is my budget? What kinds of adoption costs can I afford? Does my company have any programs to support employees who adopt?

- Would I feel comfortable parenting an older child? Am I ready for the additional challenges that come with a child who's been in the foster system for a while? How will I educate myself about these issues?

- Am I prepared to handle some level of disability in parenting a child? What extent of disability would I be comfortable with?

- How soon do I hope to bring home a child?

The Physician Letter

Before we talk more about what kind of adoption might be right for you, let's talk about your "golden ticket" for any kind of adoption: your doctor's letter.

All prospective adoptive parents, no matter how they plan to adopt, must go through a process called the home study, where

a social worker or other professional visits your home and inter-
views you and your partner (and anyone else who lives with
you) about your lives, your parenting philosophies, and all kinds
of other nitty-gritty details that help the adoption professional
decide if you're a safe person to entrust with the life of a child.
Usually, going from the beginning of a home study to the point
at which you get officially approved to adopt can take anywhere
from a month to six months or more; if you're adopting from foster care, you will likely also have to go through a series of classes
before you can be approved to adopt. (Some domestic adoption
agencies require classes as well, but most do not.)

Usually, by the time you get your home study approved, you've
already decided on what kind of adoption to pursue—because the
home study process is generally supervised by the agency you'll be
adopting through, by an independent licensed home study agency
or social worker if you're using an attorney, or by the state itself if
you're adopting from foster care. But since the doctor's letter is so
important to getting approved for adoption, we'll talk about what
it needs to say *before* we talk about how you choose an adoption
professional and move forward with the kind of adoption you
think is best for you.

One part of every home study is the medical form. It differs
from state to state and program to program, but pretty much all
home studies ask whether you have had a life-threatening illness
such as cancer.

First rule: *Don't lie*. If it comes out that you've lied in your
home study—about a cancer history or anything else—it can
completely put an end to your chances for adopting. And most of
the time, you will have to get a doctor to either fill out a medical
history form or sign off on the one you've filled out, so it's not as
if you can leave this information out or expect your doctor to do
so. Answer the Big C question completely and truthfully. For
example, you could write: "Successfully treated for testicular cancer

in 2005. My physician states that there is no evidence of any remaining cancer and that my life expectancy is normal."

But what you really need is your doctor to say that him- or herself. That gives you the best chance of having your home study approved and of having an agency give you the go-ahead to adopt. Don't just hand your doctor the form and ask that it be filled out; tell your doctor what you need it to say. If the form is general and brief (some are), ask your doctor to write a more detailed letter.

"Letters from doctors are a big challenge," says Beth Friedberg, associate director of international adoptions at Spence-Chapin in New York, a highly respected adoption agency that oversees both domestic and international adoptions. "Many times, doctors will write a very cursory letter, and we have to keep asking for more details. You want a very, very supportive letter from a doctor, explaining your diagnosis, how you were treated, and how you responded."

Make sure your doctor doesn't write the letter as if he or she is writing to another doctor. The people at adoption agencies in the United States, and adoption programs in other countries, are professionals, but they're not doctors. Don't give them jargon. The key words that most agencies will look for are "cancer free" and "normal life expectancy."

"It's best if the doctor can state that you have a normal life span, that the cancer has been fully treated and is not expected to recur, and that you are fully able to parent a child," says Vicki Peterson, executive director of external affairs for Wide Horizons for Children (WHFC), an agency with offices on the East Coast that handles both domestic and international adoptions. "It helps if [doctors] can include any statistics that they have that can support that, depending on the type of cancer and response to treatment. No doctor can guarantee anything, but the stronger [doctors] can be in terms of their expectations, the better."

Many doctors, particularly oncologists, are so busy that requests to sign forms and write letters can fall through the cracks. One way to make sure you get the letter you need promptly is to draft it yourself and save it to a flash or thumb drive. Then bring it along to your next appointment, and go over the letter with your doctor then and there. He or she can make corrections, print it out on letterhead, and sign the letter for you to take along with you.

What if you had cancer when you were fifteen, and now you're thirty-five and want to adopt? Do you still need to disclose that twenty-year-old diagnosis, even if the cancer hasn't made a peep since then? Talk with your doctor, says Peterson. "If he or she feels it's an important part of your medical history and must go on the report [he or she is] going to fill out, you need to know that," she says. "If it's something that happened in childhood, long ago, and hasn't recurred since then, it's probably a medical decision rather than an agency decision to include it. But if there's any chance at all it could show up in your home study in some other way, you don't want to leave it out and then have it surprise you."

If you get that "golden ticket"—a good doctor's letter—and you're at least a year out from cancer treatment (the precise length of time depends on what agency you're working with and what countries you're considering adopting from, if you go the international route), it's likely that your home study will be approved. Assuming, that is, that you don't have any other red flags. "We don't just look at health in a vacuum," says Friedberg. "The other parts of your life will be looked at as strengths or problems as well, by the agency, the state, and/or the country you're adopting from."

Private Domestic Adoption

Today, a lot of cancer survivors who choose adoption are opting to pursue private domestic adoption, either using an agency or an attorney. At the time of this writing, at least, it's much easier for a cancer survivor to adopt domestically than internationally. This doesn't mean you *can't* adopt internationally; it just means that fewer countries than in the past are open to approving adoptions for people with a cancer history. (More on that in "Country Codes: International Adoption," page 115.)

So, if you decide that domestic adoption is right for you, how do you move forward? How do you choose an agency or attorney? How do you get "matched" with an expectant mother considering adoption? And when and how do you bring up your cancer history with her? Or do you?

Finding a good adoption agency, or good adoption attorney, is a lot like finding a good apple in a huge bin at the grocery store. A lot of them look good on the surface, but when you turn them over, there are worms, bruises, brown spots, and other flaws. The problem is that it's a lot easier to inspect an apple at the supermarket than it is to get the inside scoop on adoption agencies or attorneys. It's important to make sure that your agency has its state license and to check out whether or not it has any complaints with the Better Business Bureau, but those are bare minimums. Similarly, your adoption attorney should be a member in good standing of the American Academy of Adoption Attorneys (Quad-A), but that alone won't tell you if you're dealing with a reputable professional.

All I can say is, take your time and do your homework—a *lot* of homework. Start by making a list of agencies or attorneys you're interested in. To get the names of agencies or attorneys who work in your state, search the online databases provided by *Adoptive Families* magazine in their Adoption Guide website:

www.theadoptionguide.com/process/finding-an-agency

www.theadoptionguide.com/process/finding-an-attorney

You can also mine theadoptionguide.com for a lot of other key resources in your agency or attorney search, including essential questions to ask any agency or attorney before signing on with them, and other sources of information for getting the scoop on agencies or attorneys you're considering.

One good source for feedback on particular adoption agencies is the Yahoo mailing list Adoption Agency Research (http://groups.yahoo.com/group/Adoption_Agency_Research/). Technically, it's focused on international adoption, but as it's evolved, there's been a lot of discussion about agencies that are involved with domestic adoptions as well (and many agencies do both). There are also agency reviews online at adoptionagencyratings.com, although it can be a bit hard to search. The Evan B. Donaldson Institute (www.adoptioninstitute.org) doesn't provide specific guidelines or questions for choosing an agency, but the wealth of resources on issues like transracial adoption, ethics and adoption, open adoption, and more make this an important stop in your adoption journey and can give you insights into what you do and *don't* want in an agency.

One question that's not on many standard lists of "what to ask an agency," not surprisingly, is "What is your policy on working with cancer survivors?" Technically, the Americans with Disabilities Act (ADA) prevents domestic adoption agencies from establishing blanket policies to screen out cancer survivors. Madelyn Freundlich of the Evan B. Donaldson Adoption Institute writes, "The law . . . requires individualized assessments based on actual risks and the use of reasonable judgment, based on current medical knowledge or on the best available objective evidence, in determining the risks involved and the actual abilities and disabilities of the individual." (Read more here: www.adoptioninstitute.org/policy/ada.html.)

But ADA or no ADA, when I first started calling adoption agencies, literally within a month or so of my breast cancer diagnosis, I expected most of them to hang up on me or at least put me off with vague politeness. Much to my surprise, not a single agency I spoke with said they would not work with cancer survivors or that they required some long posttreatment cancer-free period of three or more years. Five years later, interviewing agencies for this book, their responses were much the same. Most reputable adoption agencies will work with cancer survivors, although each one may have slightly different requirements for how long you need to have been cancer free before beginning the process.

One domestic adoption agency that's particularly cancer friendly is Abrazo, which is based in Texas but works with families all over the United States. That's because executive director Elizabeth Jurenovich is herself a breast cancer survivor. "Over the years, we've worked with a number of families where the adoptive father or adoptive mother has survived cancer, and we've found them to be wonderful parents," Jurenovich says. Abrazo usually asks prospective adoptive parents to wait a full year after completing treatment before beginning the process. "I think there's not just a physical, but an emotional healing that has to go on after dealing with cancer—just as with infertility. Our program does require documented infertility to adopt, and families coming out of the infertility treatment process are also asked to wait at least six months after concluding treatment before starting the adoption process."

The Cradle, an Illinois agency, takes a more case-by-case approach. "What we're looking for is completion of treatment. We've had people come to us who wanted to start the adoption process while in treatment, and we've asked them to wait until they've completed it, because we know that active cancer treatment takes a physical and emotional toll on you and your family," says Linda Hagemann, director of social work. "But there's a lot of research, reading, and preparing you can do during that time. And after that, we're really not looking for any specific length of time that someone is postcancer, but more what's involved in staying healthy, and treating it as any other medical condition."

(Hagemann notes that follow-up treatments—like a five-year Tamoxifen regimen after initial breast cancer treatment—wouldn't prevent someone from starting the adoption process with The Cradle.)

It's difficult to create a comprehensive list of cancer-friendly domestic adoption agencies and their policies, but what follows is a short list of nine agencies that have either directly told me that they work with cancer survivors or that have been used by other cancer survivors to adopt. Mentioning an agency on this list doesn't mean I do or do not endorse the agency, just that I know that they work with cancer survivors. (In other words, check them out yourself!) Many, but not all, of these agencies work with adoptive parents throughout the country, not just those in their state or region.

- Adoptions from the Heart, New Jersey and Pennsylvania
- Alliance for Children, Massachusetts
- Children's Home and Family Services, Minnesota
- The Cradle, Illinois
- Full Circle, Massachusetts
- Homestudies and Adoption Placement Services (HAPS), New Jersey
- Spence-Chapin, New York
- WACAP, Washington (their domestic program only places older children from foster care or African-American infants)
- Wide Horizons for Children (multiple locations on the East Coast)

Attorneys are usually even more flexible when it comes to working with cancer survivors. Many cancer survivors I know have adopted using an attorney and have had good experiences. Scott Greenberg and his wife, Rachel—you read about their inability to conceive using banked sperm in chapter 2—eventually decided to go this route after first signing up with a small, semiprivate California agency.

"Within a week after hiring our attorney, we got a phone call about two situations. In the first one, the baby had already been born and the birth mom hadn't picked us yet, but the attorney thought she would," Scott recalls. "In the second situation, the woman was pregnant and had picked us, and would be ready to sign papers when the baby was born. We decided to hold out for the baby who was already born and hope that the mom would pick us, and she did. And that was our son, Bailey—he's seven now." The Greenbergs went through a similar process to adopt daughter Peyton two-and-a-half years later.

Courtney Zinzser, also in California, used private attorneys to adopt three times. She'd been a single mom when initially diagnosed with breast cancer in 1996 at thirty-three. A year later, when the cancer returned, she managed to freeze just one embryo using donor sperm before starting chemotherapy. But she feared trying to get pregnant again after breast cancer, especially since hers was the kind fed by hormones (*hormone receptor positive*). Courtney initially considered using a surrogate but eventually ruled that out too.

As Courtney began to focus on adoption, she had some specific concerns. "I'm a special needs teacher and deal with special needs kids all day, so I felt like I couldn't handle having a special needs child at home too," says Zinzser, founder of Pink Wings 4 Breast Cancer. "I wanted domestic newborn adoption. I actually wanted twins. For months we heard nothing from our attorney, and I was getting really frustrated. Then, within two weeks, we heard from two different people—a friend of a friend, and one of the patients of my sister, who's a pediatrician—that they were looking to place babies for adoption. Both girls, both due in June."

Although some agencies caution against "artificial twinning," Courtney wanted to adopt both girls. "We were ready for two, but we thought it would probably turn out that one wouldn't go through," she says. She told one of the prospective birth moms right away about the other one, and waited a little to tell the other—but both were comfortable with the situation. Courtney's daughters, Sage and Sienna, were born within two weeks of each other.

A few years later, Courtney felt ready to adopt again. "I always wanted the Brady Bunch," she says. She went through one heartbreaking situation in which the birth mother of one of her daughters insisted that she wanted Courtney to adopt the new baby she was carrying, only to decide to parent after giving birth. Several weeks later, Courtney's attorney called her with news of a baby being born that same day. "'He's adorable, and they picked you—come in and see him tomorrow,' she said. That's how we found out about our little guy, Slayton, who's now four."

Pick Me! Pick Me!—Domestic Adoption

If you're adopting domestically, chances are pretty good that the birth mother will play some role in choosing you to adopt her child—as happened for Scott Greenberg and his wife. There are still quite a few cases in which women either tell the agency to choose adoptive parents for them, or relinquish the baby to an agency at the hospital after birth and don't want to be involved in the process at all. But that's less and less common today, so it's pretty likely that at some point, you'll need to convince a woman considering adoption that you are the right family for her baby.

Once you've signed on with your agency or attorney, the next step is usually to put together a profile of your family. Sometimes this is a one-page letter with a few photos, sometimes it's a multipage document or scrapbook. Either way, it's the next point in the journey where you will probably wonder, "What do I do about the cancer thing?"

Deciding when to disclose your cancer history to a woman who's considering you to adopt her child is kind of like deciding when to tell a new boyfriend you've had a mastectomy. The first date? Maybe too soon. Any time later? Maybe too late. It feels like there's no "good time" to make a big disclosure like that. But that's not a good reason to conceal it altogether.

Scott Greenberg took the plunge right away. "I knew my cancer would have to make its way into the profile that the birth mom would read," he recalls. "If you're concerned about who's going to raise your kid, do you want to give it to some guy who might die of cancer? There haven't been too many occasions where I felt 'disabled' or 'tainted' from the cancer, but I did then."

Now a professional motivational speaker, Scott decided to make something most people would perceive as a weakness into a strength. In their profile, the couple wrote, "Scott survived cancer as a young man, and it inspired him to become a motivational speaker to help other people overcome problems in their own lives."

"I basically explained that because of what I'd been through, I could better understand adversity," he says. "I was hoping that a birth mom would connect with that and think that maybe I could help their child become a stronger person."

Scott took exactly the right approach, says The Cradle's Linda Hagemann. "We do ask families to put medical conditions in their profile," she explains. "We practice open adoption, and as part of forming a relationship and disclosing backgrounds to each other, we ask adoptive parents to be honest about health conditions just as they want birth parents to be honest."

Like Scott, says Hagemann, you should position your cancer experience as positively as possible: "This was a challenge we faced a few years ago, but it's brought us closer together and helped make us stronger and be more resolved about our desire to be parents." Of course, you'll want to include information that the cancer has been successfully treated and you have a favorable prognosis. "Just a couple of sentences about it, and then in a meeting you could talk more," says Hagemann. "Introducing it in a letter ensures that the mother isn't caught off guard with the information later."

Many adoption professionals say that women considering adoption react with surprising equanimity to the idea that the adoptive parents they're considering have cancer in their background. "Most of the moms we work with, they're not strangers to hard knocks, to life. They realize that life has its ups and downs and they're pretty realistic about it," says Hagemann. "I don't think they're under any illusion that adoption is just going to be all perfection. We've had families with prior marriages, families with a health issue or something difficult in their background, parents who are recovering alcoholics. Birth parents typically are grateful for the honesty and the fact that this is somebody who has been successful in dealing with a challenge."

That's not to say that families with a cancer history haven't sometimes been skipped over for that reason. But Hagemann says that most of the time, prospective birth parents are looking for specific things in a family: a particular religious background, a home in the country or in the city, a stay-at-home parent, a childless couple or older siblings, particular educational opportunities. In other words, you're just as likely to be chosen, or not chosen, because of how many other kids you have as because you had thyroid cancer three years ago. It's about the whole you, not just the "cancer you."

What if you're not comfortable with putting your cancer diagnosis in the profile? Is it okay to wait until a prospective birth mom shows interest in you and share the information as you're getting to know each other? That's fine, says Abrazo's Elizabeth Jurenovich—as long as you do use the "C word" before the expectant mom has made any commitments to you. "There are a whole host of details about a family that are not necessarily appropriate for a profile. To some extent it depends on how relevant it is to who you are as a couple and how recent it is," she says. "But remember that birth parents are expected to be truthful and forthright, and we owe them the same level of honesty."

When we adopted our daughter in 2006, I was less than two years out from my 2004 cancer diagnosis. We'd just been on the classic adoption roller coaster: two failed matches with one agency, including one where we'd flown hundreds of miles to await the birth only to find out after the baby was born that her mom decided to parent—a few weeks before Christmas. This was followed by a bad "breakup" with that agency, and then a situation with an unscrupulous lawyer who promoted a match with an expectant seventeen-year-old, only to do a 180 when our own lawyer told her that her fees were beyond the limits allowed by New Jersey law. The other attorney then revealed that the girl's mother was supposedly very leery of my cancer history and had been planning to put the kibosh on the match anyway.

So with our second agency, I shied away from putting anything about my cancer diagnosis in writing. It wasn't in our profile, and it wasn't in the letter we wrote directly to our daughter's birth mother, when the agency told us there was a young woman in Georgia due in a month who wanted to hear more about us.

Instead, I think we took the coward's way out. We told K. about my cancer history on a visit to her hometown, during dinner at a big, loud, festive Mexican restaurant. I didn't exactly mumble, "GreatnachospassthesalsabythewayIhadcancer," but I didn't say, "Look, there's something important you should know," either. I tried to slip it into the conversation as unobtrusively as possible while still being able to tell myself that I'd told her. As it turned out, she really didn't have much of a concern about it—but I don't like how we handled it. If we had it to do over again, we *would* have put the cancer history in our profile because I think that Linda Hagemann is right on all counts. Prospective adoptive parents owe the people who are going to entrust them with their children the whole truth, and we often sell people short. I believe having battled cancer makes me a stronger person and a better mom, so why not say that in a profile?

Country Codes: International Adoption

If you choose to adopt from another country, your big question won't be "How do I explain my cancer history in a profile for a woman considering adoption to read?" Instead, it will be, "What country or countries will allow me to adopt as a cancer survivor?" Because although you may pass a home study done by your adoption agency, that doesn't mean that you will be approved by the authorities of the country you wish to adopt from. Each country has its own policies about what kind of health history they're willing to consider in prospective adoption parents—policies that aren't always quite clear, but that U.S. adoption agencies have little, if any ability to change.

If I were writing this book six or seven years ago, this section would be much different. When I was diagnosed with breast cancer in 2004 and made the conscious decision to forego fertility preservation, I almost immediately began exploring adoption possibilities, both international and domestic. At that time, agencies I spoke with reassured me that there were a number of cancer-friendly countries, chief among them being China and Guatemala.

That was then; this is now. Today, the picture has changed drastically. "In general, most countries have become more restrictive about what mental and physical health conditions they will accept in adoptive parents," says WHFC's Vicki Peterson.

Several years ago, China introduced restrictive new guidelines as to who can adopt from that country; one of the new requirements is that if you've ever been diagnosed with cancer, you must be at least ten years cancer free. Even for prospective adoptive parents with no health issues at all, the wait for Chinese adoptions has slowed to such a trickle that, as a practical matter, it makes almost no sense to start the process of adopting from China today unless you are open to adopting a child with significant special needs—or you're fine with waiting four, five, or more years to bring home your child.

Adoptions from Guatemala to the United States, meanwhile, have been shut down entirely since the United States became a signatory to the Hague Adoption Convention, an intercountry agreement designed to protect child trafficking and exploitation and ensure that adoptions are in the best interests of the children involved. Guatemala is technically a signatory to the Hague Convention, but there have been major concerns raised about the ethics of adoption practices in Guatemala, and the United States has suspended all adoptions from that country until it achieves compliance with the Convention's requirements. Guatemalan adoptions may reopen someday, but it's unlikely to be very soon.

Dawn Davenport, who writes the Creating a Family adoption blog, has called the current situation a "perfect storm" of international adoption delays, not just for cancer survivors but for everyone. With Guatemala (and Vietnam) shutting down to U.S. adoptions, and many people turning away from China due to its delays and restrictions, the timeline for adoptions from other countries—like Russia and Ethiopia—is slowing down as more prospective adoptive parents seek out these programs.

So where does that leave you as a cancer survivor? When I first started thinking about this book, I expected to include a clear and specific chart listing which countries were cancer friendly and which were not. But it's more complicated than that. The problem is that the international adoption picture is an ever-changing one. Some countries close down to international adoptions; others open or reopen; still others change their rules.

"Every country has a different policy on how long ago a cancer history needs to be," says Jessica Palmer, social work coordinator with Holt International, one of the best-known international agencies. "I can keep track of what countries say when I ask something about a client's cancer history on a case-by-case basis, and then I can ask a week later and get a different answer. It's almost impossible to have a hard-and-fast rule."

So I have a chart for you—but it's a lot vaguer than I wanted it to be. This chart includes a list of most of the countries from which U.S. citizens can currently adopt, the children generally available for adoption, the countries' basic requirements of adoptive parents (age requirements, income, etc.), their stance on a cancer history and other health issues, and some of the larger and better-known agencies that currently work in those countries. This is *not* an exhaustive chart of all the requirements, issues, paperwork, travel required, and timeline for each country—just basic info that should give you an idea of whether you'd want to explore a particular country further. The information comes from the State Department's public information on adoption from these countries, as well as the public websites of reputable agencies working in these countries. Just keep in mind that a lot can change very fast in international adoption, so use this information only as a jumping-off point, and verify everything you read here with current State Department and agency information!

Burundi

Burundi adoptions to the United States are relatively new, and programs are in development at a couple of major American agencies. Some other pilot programs are in different stages at various agencies as well, in countries including the Democratic Republic of Congo, Lesotho, and Rwanda. Pilot programs such as these can often move very quickly; they can also shut down just as quickly. While they may be more open to cancer survivors, they may also be more vulnerable to ethical violations, so proceed with your eyes wide open.

REQUIREMENTS The program is open to married couples and heterosexual women, ages thirty to fifty-five. Couples should have been married and living together for at least five years prior to beginning the process.

CHILDREN Children are older infants to teenagers. They are cared for in private orphanages.

CANCER? The program asks for no major medical history. So early on with a new program, it's hard to know how a cancer history will be viewed, but adoption professionals recommend presenting a cancer history in context, as part of a family's overall dossier, for the most favorable case-by-case consideration.

AGENCIES Wide Horizons for Children

China

Practically speaking, China has become almost exclusively a special-needs program for any new adoption applicants. The new requirements instituted in 2007, plus a general slowdown of the process, means that there is usually a more than three-year wait from beginning the process to bringing a child home. U.S. adoptions from China are down significantly from their peak of more than 7,000 in 2004 to just under 5,500 in 2007.

REQUIREMENTS Parents must be a legally married heterosexual couple, ages thirty to forty-nine, with no more than four children already in the household and an income of at least $10,000 per family member (including the child to be adopted).

CHILDREN Children are at least seven months old at time of placement, usually over a year. There are more girls than boys. Children awaiting adoption live in Chinese orphanages.

CANCER? In most cases, China requires that you be ten years cancer free before you can adopt. But if you are willing to adopt a child of three or older with significant special needs, such as a heart defect, you may be able to get a medical exemption. Such adoptions can also sometimes move much more quickly.

AGENCIES Alliance for Children, Children's Home Society and Family Services, Holt, Spence-Chapin, WACAP, Wide Horizons for Children

Colombia

Colombian adoptions are among the more stable and long-standing adoption programs offered by many U.S. adoption agencies today.

REQUIREMENTS Parents must be married and each should be between twenty-five and thirty-eight years old to adopt babies and younger children. Older parents and single men and women may adopt older children and those with special needs and must have no more than two children already at home.

CHILDREN About half of all children placed from Colombia are under one year of age. The wait is usually about eighteen months to three years, with longer time frames for younger infants. Children live in both private orphanages and foster care.

CANCER? Eligibility is limited to applicants without physical health issues that impair their daily lives or life span. Colombia tends to be conservative in its health requirements, but depending on the type of cancer and long-term prognosis, they may be willing to consider cancer survivors on a case-by-case basis.

AGENCIES Alliance for Children, Children's Home Society and Family Services, Spence-Chapin, Wide Horizons for Children

Ethiopia

In 2006, 731 immigrant visas for adoption were issued to children from Ethiopia; this number nearly tripled, to 2,277, by 2009. The sharp spike in interest in Ethiopian adoption has also led to concerns about ethics and accountability, as often happens when a country becomes "popular" for adoptions, so choose your agency carefully. Some agencies say that cancer survivors meet with more understanding in Ethiopian adoptions; others have a specific five-year cancer-free rule for Ethiopia. As of this writing, that is a requirement of some agencies, not the country itself, and I know of multiple cancer survivors who have completed Ethiopian adoptions well before reaching the "five-year cancer-free" mark.

REQUIREMENTS Parents should be couples married at least one year, both over twenty-five and under fifty-six, with no more than a fifty-year age difference between youngest parent and child.

CHILDREN Children are infants, toddlers, children, and sibling groups. You must be open to a child up to thirty-six months of age; some babies do arrive home as young as six months, but this is rare. Children awaiting adoption live in group care centers.

CANCER? It is required that you have no chronic medical conditions that would impact the parenting of a child. Conditions like cancer are considered on a case-by-case basis; at present, most agencies will tell you that at this time, Ethiopia is one of the best prospects for cancer survivors considering international adoption.

AGENCIES Alliance for Children, Children's Home Society and Family Services, Holt, Spence-Chapin, Wide Horizons for Children, WACAP

Guatemala

All U.S. adoption programs in Guatemala are suspended indefinitely. Guatemala is not a signatory to the Hague Adoption Convention.

Haiti

The devastating earthquake of January 2010 left Haitian adoption programs in turmoil. Many adoptions were expedited for children already in the process of being adopted, but much of the adoption system in place in Haiti—staff, records, facilities—was lost in the earthquake. In May 2010, Haiti's adoption authority began accepting new applications for children who either were documented as orphans before the quake or had been formally relinquished by their birth parents since January 12. But most U.S. agencies continue to proceed with caution in Haiti.

India

The process for adopting from India can be volatile, and many agencies that work in India encourage adoptive families to "double apply" or have a backup country in the event that the process is disrupted.

REQUIREMENTS Parents should be couples aged twenty-eight to forty, with no more than fifteen years' age difference between them. There should be at least twenty-one and no more than forty-five years between parent and child. If at least one parent is not of documented Indian heritage/citizenship status (nonresident Indian or Overseas Citizen of India), then you will be matched with a child of thirty-six months or older. Sometimes India will consider single women up to age forty-five who have not been married previously.

CHILDREN Children are toddlers, school-aged children, and sibling groups.

CANCER? India requires adoptive parents to have no serious health concerns. As with other countries that have broad statements like this, cancer survivors may be able to adopt from India on a case-by-case basis.

AGENCIES Children's Home Society and Family Services, Wide Horizons for Children

Kazakhstan

Kazakhstan temporarily put adoptions to the United States on hold in 2008, with little explanation, but has recently begun to process them again. Some agencies are working again in Kazakhstan on a pilot basis. WACAP and Wide Horizons are among those agencies.

REQUIREMENTS Parent(s) should be married couples and single women no more than forty-five years of age.

CHILDREN Children are usually between six months and three years old at the time of referral, but children up to fifteen years old need families. They generally reside in "baby homes" (orphanages) and represent a variety of ethnicities, including Asian, Eurasian, and Caucasian.

CANCER? WACAP reports that Kazakhstan is one of the countries that it considers "more flexible" on cancer than others.

AGENCIES Alliance for Children, WACAP, Wide Horizons for Children

Korea

Korea has some of the most strict and specific standards for adoptive parents of any country. There are also far fewer agencies working in Korea than in many other countries; they are very restrictive as to whom they work with. Some agencies have slowed down their Korea adoption processes lately.

REQUIREMENTS Parents should be couples over twenty-five and under forty-three at time of submission, married at least three years. There should be no more than five children (including the prospective adopted child) under eighteen in the family. There are strict health requirements, including a BMI of less than 30.

CHILDREN Children are infants of both genders, and there are many more boys than girls. They usually arrive home between eight and twelve months of age and live in small nurseries before entering foster care while awaiting adoption.

CANCER? Korea generally requires a five-year cancer-free period before cancer survivors can adopt. If you've cleared the five-year hurdle, though, the process is otherwise considered to be fairly smooth and predictable.

AGENCIES Children's Home Society and Family Services, Holt, Spence-Chapin, WACAP (only in certain states), Wide Horizons for Children

Nepal

As of August 2010, the United States has suspended adoption from Nepal because of concerns about unreliable and fabricated documents. (Technically, the suspension applies only to adoptions of children reported abandoned, but in practice, this applies to all Nepali adoptions.) It's unknown when and whether these adoptions will resume.

Philippines

Wide Horizons for Children calls the Philippine adoption program one of its most stable. All adoptions in the Philippines are overseen by a government body, the Intercountry Adoption Board.

REQUIREMENTS Parent(s) should be couples with a formal legal relationship of at least three years, ages twenty-seven to forty-five. Parents over forty-five may adopt a slightly older child. Single applicants are allowed to adopt children six or older or with special needs. Same-gender couples may not adopt from the Philippines. Documented infertility is required.

CHILDREN As of May 1, 2009, the Philippines instituted a temporary moratorium on the adoption of children aged two and younger, because of a large backlog of prospective adoptive parents awaiting adoption of babies and young toddlers. Adoptions of children aged three and older are still proceeding. Preschool and school-aged children, and sibling groups are available for adoption; they live in both foster care and orphanage settings.

CANCER? Parents should have no serious medical issues—but the requirements do not specify whether there is a problem with medical issues, such as cancer, that have been successfully treated in the past. Cancer is generally handled on a case-by-case basis.

AGENCIES Holt, Wide Horizons for Children

Russia

Almost everyone has heard of the case of seven-year-old Artyom Savelyev, who was returned to Russia on a plane by himself in April 2010, after his adoptive mother claimed she could no longer parent him. This case has thrown Russian adoptions to the United States into turmoil. These adoptions are apparently still proceeding, and American and Russian officials have reached accord on an adoption pact. Russia's parliament has rejected a motion to halt all American adoptions. But Russian officials themselves differ on whether they want to suspend adoptions to the United States or allow the program to continue. This is definitely a "stay tuned" matter that can change day by day. At the end of July 2010, the Joint Council on International Children's Services reported that although the status hasn't officially changed, prospective adoptive parents should be prepared for possible delays.

REQUIREMENTS Parent(s) should be couples married at least one year, and single women. Russia prefers no more than forty-five years between the youngest parent and child.

CHILDREN Children are both genders and all ages; there are more boys than girls. Many parents bring home toddlers under two, but adoption of infants under one year is almost unheard of. Children generally live in orphanages, but foster care is becoming more available.

CANCER? Some agencies consider Russia very cancer friendly, while others say just the opposite. A lot depends on the region or regions in which the agency works. In general, Russia considers health issues like a cancer history on a case-by-case basis. Some regions may require the parent with a cancer history to have a medical examination in Russia.

AGENCIES Alliance for Children, Children's Home Society and Family Services, Holt, Spence-Chapin, WACAP, Wide Horizons for Children

Rwanda

Rwanda, one of the newest international adoption pilot programs in the United States, has been temporarily suspended while they work on implementing the Hague process. As with all newer and pilot programs, it's still hard to predict exactly how the process will work in the future.

REQUIREMENTS Parent(s) should be couples married at least five years with no more than one divorce each, aged thirty to fifty, or single, heterosexual females aged thirty-five to fifty. You can have no more than two children in the home already.

CHILDREN Children are boys and girls of all ages, especially infants to two years.

CANCER? Applicants should have no major medical history. It's hard to know exactly how Rwanda's new pilot program will respond to parents with a cancer history, but some adoption professionals think that, like Ethiopia, they will be more flexible.

AGENCIES Wide Horizons for Children

Taiwan

Taiwan essentially has two adoption programs: one for parents interested in adopting a non–special needs baby or young child, and the other for those open to special needs or older children. Some agencies offer programs in which the birth parents select the adoptive parents, although traditional closed adoptions are also available. Taiwan requires adoptive parents to complete post-placement reports for five years.

REQUIREMENTS Applicants must be between twenty-five and fifty-five years of age and at least twenty years older than the child they wish to adopt. Applicants over forty will be considered for older children and those with special needs. There can be no more than three children already in the home; you may only have one child if you want to adopt a healthy child under five.

CHILDREN Most children are at least a year old when they come home, and many have some minor to significant special needs.

CANCER? Taiwan requires that applicants be in good mental and physical health, but what exactly that may mean is vague. WHFC's Vicki Peterson suggests that the country may be willing to work with applicants who are at least two years out from successful treatment.

AGENCIES Alliance for Children, Wide Horizons for Children

Vietnam

Adoptions from Vietnam to the United States were shut down in 2005, reopened in 2006, and shut down again in 2008 after allegations of corruption. While open, the Vietnam adoption process was considered fairly welcoming for cancer survivors, but there's no way to know when things will start up again.

Here are some tips for thinking about adopting internationally as a cancer survivors:

1. **Look for a well-known agency with a long track record in international adoption.** This is important for any prospective adoptive parents, but even more so for cancer survivors, who may be more vulnerable to the come-on tactics of more fly-by-night agencies. Here is a short list of some well-known agencies with long track records, who have told me that they work with cancer survivor:

   Adoption Associates, Michigan

   Alliance for Children, Massachusetts

   Children's Home Society and Family Services, Minnesota

Holt International, Oregon

Spence-Chapin, New York

WACAP, Oregon

Wide Horizons for Children, multiple East Coast offices

2. **Make sure that the agency works with multiple countries—** and, as long as it's a reputable and ethical agency, the more the better. That way, if one country changes its policies, you don't have to find an entirely new agency in order to begin the adoption process from a different country. In fact, it might not be a bad idea to consider an agency that has both domestic and international programs, giving you as much flexibility as possible should circumstances change.

3. **Do not accept as gospel the word of the first agency (or second, or third) you speak with as to whether you can adopt from a particular country.** Different agencies may work in different regions of a particular country and with different orphanages or other entities in the adoption process. One agency may be able to help you adopt as a cancer survivor from a reputedly "cancer-unfriendly" country because the agency works in a region where the policies vary somewhat. "Some countries have a centralized system, where the government states some eligibility guidelines for adoptive parents," explains Spence-Chapin's Beth Friedberg. "Sometimes the guidelines are explicit, sometimes they're implicit, and sometimes there's flexibility and sometimes there isn't. You may contact one agency that says they can't work with you for X country, and then another agency that says they know that one part of the country is more flexible than others."

4. **Know what kinds of questions to ask.** If an agency says they can't work with you as a cancer survivor to adopt

from X country, ask "Is this the practice of your agency or the country? Is it national or regional? Where might there be some flexibility?" This doesn't mean you should never take no for an answer, but the right questions can help you understand if something is worth pursuing further.

5. **Keep good records.** As you start calling agencies, set up a spreadsheet and write down what each of them tells you about the specific cancer policies of a particular country and how they work in each country.

6. **Think seriously about what kind of situation you are prepared to accept.** You will significantly increase your chances of being able to adopt internationally if you're open to adopting an older child or a child with special needs. Remember that special needs in some countries may mean nothing more than cleft lips or palates, missing fingers, major birthmarks, or even just being older. Many of these issues are considered very significant in some countries but are easily correctable in the United States. But only consider special needs adoption if you are clear about what kinds of situations you will and will not accept and have educated yourself about what those special needs will really mean for your family and what you need to do to prepare to bring home a child with these specific needs.

7. **Think about what kinds of risks you're prepared to take.** "Some people who survive cancer feel more resourceful, like they have new strength and new coping strategies," says Friedberg. "Others may come in feeling really depleted, emotionally, financially, or both, and not want to put themselves out there again. They want something that's more predictable." Of course, the reality is that adoption is never predictable, and even the most "stable" country for adoptions may not turn out to be so stable after all. "When we

want something really badly, we want to go to what feels like it has the path of least resistance. You want a program that will bring your child home ASAP. But programs change all the time. You have to realize that the possibility for change is greater than anything."

8. **Remember that cancer is only part of your picture.** You may have other aspects to your life that are strong positives for the country you want to adopt from—a particular religious tradition, a long and stable marriage, lots of extended family support. On the other hand, there may be other "red flags" in your background. Some countries consider any past antidepressant use or treatment for mental health issues to be a problem, for example—even though it may be hardly surprising or unusual that someone might take antidepressants for a while during cancer treatment!

9. **Keep trying!** As you'll learn from the next story, doors that you think will remain closed might suddenly decide to swing open.

Even countries that seem entirely closed off to cancer survivors may not always be so unwelcoming. Anne Eastbourne (names of this family changed upon request) had adopted her daughter Jie Jie from China in February 2007, when the little girl was four and a half. She'd been home just eight months when Anne was diagnosed with stage I breast cancer. After a lumpectomy, four rounds of chemotherapy, and radiation, Anne and her husband, Mike, were ready to adopt again.

"Because our daughter was older coming home, we feel that God gave us the ability to care for older children, and we very much want to adopt older kids," Anne says. "We knew that China had changed their rules in May 2007 and was much more strict about a cancer history, so we figured they were out. We called at least thirty agencies, and I think we looked at every country in the world."

The family went through a changing list of countries and options—Nepal? Krygyzstan? Bulgaria? Domestic foster care? Then one day in August 2009, Jie Jie, then seven, confronted her mother. "Mommy, why aren't we adopting from China?" she asked.

"Darling, we can't," Anne answered.

"Mommy, did you try? Did you just try? Did you call China and ask them?" Jie Jie demanded.

"We had a whole long discussion about why we can't adopt from China because Mommy had cancer," Anne says. When Jie Jie wouldn't take no for an answer, Anne decided to show her the website of Chinese Children Adoption International, a large agency that posts a clear, detailed online description of the country's rules. "I go down the list and say, 'See here? Rule #7. No cancer survivors,'" she says. "But then I see that it doesn't say that anymore. It says, 'Cancer survivors on a case-by-case basis.'" (Today, CCAI's website reads, "If an applicant has a history of any cancer, please contact CCAI before completing the Application for Adoption.")

Stunned, Anne called the agency. "They told us that in just the last week, China had indicated they were open to considering cancer survivors for the waiting child program," she says. "On August 5, we submitted a request for an exception, and ten days later we got the exception straight from the medical board: we could try to adopt a child three or older with special needs, like a heart defect."

Since Jie Jie had come to them with a heart defect of her own, Anne felt more than ready for that challenge. Anne went back to the agency she'd been working with and said, "See if you can match us." The very next day, they got a phone call. "We have a referral for a four-year-old boy—would you like to look at his file?" They would. They did. And in May 2010, they traveled to China to bring home their son, then nearly five. "If it hadn't been for my daughter insisting, we would have completely given up on China," Anne says. "Keep calling and calling and do your research."

That's perfect advice, says Rebecca Carter (name changed at her request), who was diagnosed with breast cancer at the age of forty-four in 2006. Carter and her husband both had grown children from a previous marriage, but they yearned to have a baby together. They had gone through IVF and miscarriages before Rebecca's diagnosis, and they knew that after cancer and chemotherapy, adoption was probably their only chance to be parents again.

After rejecting domestic adoption, the Carters thought of Russia, where Rebecca's husband had been born. But the first few agencies they spoke with told them they couldn't adopt from Russia so soon after cancer treatment (she was just six months out when she began the process), and that when enough time had passed, they'd be too old. "When I heard a few agencies tell me it was impossible, I thought that there was no way of doing it," Rebecca says. "But then I went through the list of agencies that were accredited to work in Russia at the time and called each and every one of them. Every one had a different story."

One accredited agency, Alliance for Children, didn't just tell Rebecca a blanket policy. "They asked about my history and what my doctors thought and if I could get a positive medical report about my condition," Rebecca recalls. "It was a really detailed interview about my whole history. Then they said, okay, go ahead and submit your application. They assigned me to a region [that] is more flexible about certain things. Some regions, for example, require that you go to a doctor in Russia to be examined. We didn't have to do that."

By the end of September 2007, when Rebecca was barely a year out of treatment, they had received the referral for their son.

They traveled to Russia to meet him in November and returned to bring him home in January. "He's changed our lives. He just turned three, and he's the cutest, the sweetest," she says.

Susan Nichols, the founder of the adoption-after-cancer Yahoo email group, has adopted twice internationally after her breast cancer diagnosis in 2001. Just two years out of treatment, she and her husband started pursuing a Russian adoption to add to their family—they have a daughter, Haeli, who was then nine years old. "I did a lot of research while in treatment and met another family who'd adopted a daughter from China and three girls from Kazakhstan. Even though I got my periods back very quickly after chemo—I was thirty-one at the time—we decided that maybe adoption was our little calling."

The family chose Russia because they wanted to adopt two children at once, something that was difficult to do at the time in other countries. Susan was very careful with the way she described her cancer in documents for the Russian authorities. "I didn't say, 'cancer'—I said that I had 'a little lump.' I couldn't make the cancer who I was for the home study," she says. "Fortunately, I had a social worker who had a family member who'd had breast cancer and understood what the terms meant. She said she could write a positive home study if the doctor gave me a letter saying I was free of cancer and that I could have a reasonable chance at a normal life expectancy. So that's what he wrote. And then she called their regional connections and found a region that was open to working with someone with a history of cancer."

In December 2003, Susan and her husband brought home their two sons, Ethan and Zachary, then eighteen months and thirteen months. In the summer of 2010, they adopted two brothers from Ethiopia who are now six and eight, and shortly afterward began the process to bring home the boys' sister, whom they had just found out about. They have also adopted a teenage daughter who was their foster child for several years. "That would be six children adopted after stage 2b breast cancer, adopted from three different countries, including the U.S. foster system. They are all wonderful," Nichols says. "I rarely talk about the cancer to any adoption officials, social workers, agencies, and so on. It doesn't define who I am. It was an episode in my life."

Foster Parenting and Adoption

When people say, "There are so many children who need homes," they're generally talking about children in foster care, whether they realize it or not. Every year, about 50,000 children are adopted from foster care in the United States, while about 125,000 are still awaiting adoption. According to the Department of Health and Human Services, children in foster care are more likely to be older, members of a minority group, members of a sibling group, or survivors of abuse or neglect.

Deciding whether foster parenting is right for you—either with the goal of eventually adopting a child that you foster, or not—is a very complex question, in many ways beyond the scope of this book. There are some excellent books on foster parenting and foster-adoption listed in the Resources section at the end of this book. Here I'll give you the basics and then talk about what your prospects are to foster-adopt as a cancer survivor.

Foster parenting and foster-adoption can be very different depending on what state you live in. To become a foster parent, you must first go through a state-run process for becoming licensed, which usually includes

- Background check and fingerprinting
- Comprehensive home study
- Classroom hours
- First aid certification
- Medical clearances for all adults and children in the home

In some ways, becoming a foster parent may sound easier than successfully adopting internationally or through domestic private adoption. After all, as long as you're twenty-one and have your own income, you can often still qualify as a foster parent in most states even if you're older, single, don't own your home, already have multiple children, and/or rely on some government assistance. But there's much more to it than that.

Each state has different training requirements for foster parents, ranging from as few as six hours of classroom training to as many as forty-five. You can find more specific information about how the foster parenting process works in your state at www.adoptuskids.org. This training is important. Children who are in foster care are there for a reason; they have been separated from their birth family because the child protection authorities think their home is not a safe or appropriate environment for them. That means that they may have been abused or neglected. At minimum, they have undergone the traumatic experience of being separated from their parents. Foster parents need to be prepared to cope with the unique needs of these children and with the fact that they will be parenting under the state's supervision. That may mean regular meetings with social workers and other professionals, visits with birth parents, and not being able to make ordinary family decisions—like traveling out of state for the holidays—without clearing it with your child's caseworker or the court.

Children's Sake of Virginia, a child placing agency, suggests that you ask yourself the following questions before you decide whether or not to become a foster parent:

1. Can you provide care, protection, fun, and empathy to a child who doesn't understand you and may not give back in a way you are accustomed to?

2. Are you sure of your parenting skills but willing to learn new skills to deal with new behaviors?

3. Can you adopt good, firm boundaries right from the start while remaining secure in your ability to parent?

4. Can you love and care for a child who has come from an environment that is completely different than your own?

5. Can you care about a child and help them feel like they belong with your family while knowing that the child's placement with your family may end before you are ready?

6. Can you discipline with empathy and know that the anger a child may feel and express is not personally directed at you although it may look and feel as though it is?

7. Can you maintain an understanding that behavioral problems of any kind are often a direct result of abuse or neglect?

8. Can you measure success and failure in new and creative ways?

9. Can you work as part of a professional team while you may disagree with the process or outcome?

10. Can you tenaciously advocate for the rights of a child?

11. Can you accept a relationship with parents you might never want to know because of behavior they have expressed with the child you care for?

12. Can you remember that love and loss are sometimes very hard to do and that you have to let go when it seems impossible?

States have different names for the agencies that supervise foster care. For example, in New Jersey, it's the Department of Youth and Family Services; in Texas, it's the Department of Family and Protective Services. In many states, there are also private nonprofit agencies that work in partnership with these state agencies to license and supervise foster parents. You can find state and private foster care agencies near you by searching the Child Welfare Information Gateway's directory at www.childwelfare .gov/nfcad/.

Sometimes, it can be easier to find out about foster care opportunities in your area by talking to one of the private agencies than by calling an overworked and underfunded state agency. Google "foster care agency" and add the name of your state, and you should be able to find agencies near you.

What will the state, or the private agency, say when they find out you're a cancer survivor? In many cases, not much. States generally require that prospective foster parents be in "good physical and mental health" and not have any current medical conditions that would affect their ability to parent a child—so unless you're currently in treatment and it has substantially impaired you, you'll often find that your cancer history presents no problem at all.

In Michigan, for example, "So long as their doctor says it's okay, there isn't any restriction," says Carol Slottke, a child welfare licensing consultant at the Department of Human Services. "We have some people who are foster parents who have gone through cancer treatment and continued to foster while being treated, in fact. If there's a medical condition that arises while they're fostering, the agency can request another doctor's statement, but unless it's a major impairment, there's no problem."

Casey Family Services, a private agency that licenses foster parents in Connecticut, Maine, Massachusetts, New Hampshire, Rhode Island, and Vermont, as well as Baltimore, Maryland, is similarly flexible with cancer survivors. "The parents need not to have had a 'life-changing experience or trauma' within the past year, which I would think would include cancer," says Roye Anastasio Bourke, Casey's public affairs manager. "But if someone had gone through their final cancer treatment a little less than a year before, and had been well and functioning and able to participate in life full-time for a year, I can't imagine that they would turn anybody away. I think that the concern with our agency would be to know that the person was strong enough and felt healthy enough to parent a child. We have to consider, first and foremost, the needs of the child—many of them have been removed from their homes and have behavioral issues and attachment issues. We need to be sure a foster parent has enough support to meet these challenges."

Social workers and other foster care professionals in several other states, including North Carolina, expressed much the same sentiments. In fact, I haven't yet talked to anyone working with the foster care system in any state who has said that it might be difficult for a cancer survivor—assuming that their condition has been successfully treated—to become a foster parent or adopt through foster care.

Jim and Joy DeLaere, who had daughter Lillian and son Lincoln via IVF using sperm frozen before Jim's cancer treatment, had also long considered becoming foster parents. "Growing up I had a foster brother, and we'd heard some ads for sibling groups who needed to be adopted together. I went to an adoption conference, and the Illinois Department of Children and Family Services was there, saying how much they need foster parents," Joy recalls.

The DeLaeres went through an eighteen-month process to become foster parents—with delays not because of Jim's cancer, but because of state budget problems. "They didn't bat an eye at his cancer history," Joy says. They received their foster care license in June 2009, and in February 2010 began fostering brother-and-sister siblings, ages eleven and thirteen.

Christa Michael, a real estate agent in Georgia, was first diagnosed with breast cancer in 2004, shortly before she turned forty. She had a grown son from a previous marriage and had lost another son in infancy, and then decided after the cancer recurred that she wasn't done with parenting. Her sister's two young children, then just three months and four years old, were in need of a foster home, and Christa immediately volunteered.

"They did ask for all my medical records, but they were much less focused on the cancer than on home evaluations and drug tests," Christa says. She's since gone through additional recurrences and had a scare when a broker with a real estate company she then worked with called the child services agency because she thought Christa couldn't parent the children since she had cancer again. "I spent the next two weeks in terror with emergency hearings, fearful that they were going to come and get my kids," she says. "But eventually we resolved it." Ultimately, her sister's parental rights were terminated, and Christa finalized the children's adoption in early 2010.

She's now planning on fostering more children—two siblings, close to the ages her two are now. "No more adoptions—although I say that *now* . . ." she laughs.

Carly Chandler, who was diagnosed with stage III breast cancer in 2003, also didn't find her cancer history any barrier to foster care and adoption. Initially diagnosed when she was pregnant with her second son, Carly went through the works: an induced early delivery, chemotherapy, a double mastectomy, and eventually, a hysterectomy and oophorectomy (removal of her ovaries) when she was diagnosed with the BRCA2 mutation that increases risk for multiple gynecological cancers.

At first, her own fears about her health and her future—never mind anyone else's—kept Carly from even considering having more children. "But once I was alive for a couple of years, I realized I might stay healthy, and my husband and I started to talk about foster-adopt," she says. "That was always something we'd wanted to do, adopt. And even if I hadn't had cancer, private and overseas adoption were just too expensive. This was our only option, and that was fine. It was kind of a hard path, but private adoption can be too."

The Chandlers began going through the licensing process in Oceanside, California, where they then lived (Carly's husband is in the Marine Corps, and they have moved frequently), in February 2007. "We got licensed and got our foster son within a few weeks," she says. "We only did foster-adopt and asked to only foster children who were most likely to be adoptable." Their little boy was four months old, but as a preemie, he was more like a one-month-old. When he was almost a year old, the boy's biological mother gave birth again, and the Chandlers began fostering his little sister when she was seven months old. They recently finalized the adoptions of both children, now one and two years old.

Throughout the process, her cancer never posed an issue. "That was one of our first questions—is this going to affect anything? They said no—in fact, they'd had foster parents and adoptive parents where *both* members of the couple had had cancer," Carly says. "As long as my doctor could say I was able to take care of children twenty-four hours a day, that was pretty much it."

Recurrence During the Process

What if the cancer comes back while you're in the process of adoption? Usually, your agency will ask that you put your application on hold until your condition is stable—but it doesn't have to derail your adoption plans completely.

Pam Staples actually found out she had stage I endometrial cancer while in the process of fertility testing, when something looked "not quite right" on her ultrasound. At the time, she opted to skip a hysterectomy, still hoping to have biological children. She took a drug called Megace (megestrol) for several months, after which tests revealed the cancer had apparently been eradicated. Pam and her husband continued pursuing fertility treatments, and went from fertility drugs to intrauterine insemination to in vitro fertilization, with no success. Finally, in early 2008, they decided to pursue adoption instead.

They chose domestic adoption, thinking that lengthy overseas travel would be difficult with Pam's husband's new job. They researched agencies, talking to other people who had had cancer and to adoption attorneys in an effort to find one that was cancer friendly.

"Since my cancer was very early stage I, my doctors said, 'Don't worry, we can work around it,'" Pam says. "They were very supportive of our family-building efforts." Ultimately, the couple chose a local agency in North Carolina. "They said, 'With cancer, we work around it, we listen to what your doctor has to say.' My doctor had already said that I have a full life expectancy and I just need to continue to take follow-up measures."

But as they were making plans for their home study, in August 2008, Pam was diagnosed with thyroid cancer. That fall was grueling: she had her thyroid removed and went through a week of intensive pill-form radiation therapy, using radioactive iodine, that put her in seclusion for eight days. "I had to have at least ten feet between me and the nearest adult," she says. "All my bedsheets had to be washed separately. Our cats and dog couldn't be anywhere near me. I couldn't touch anyone else's food."

In mid-November 2008, her full body scan came back clean, and she's been cancer free ever since. "In the meantime, I was informing the agency what we were doing. They said that the key item they needed was regular updates from both my doctors while going through this process. They wanted something from my doctor that said this would not kill me, that I had a full life expectancy," Pam says. "My doctor wrote a really nice letter and included a bunch of studies on thyroid cancer and life expectancy. The agency asked for some additional information about treatments and how often I would have to go for follow-up. The home study was completed in December, and we got the formal notice of approval in January."

Eight months later, in August 2009, the agency called. There was a baby due in mid-September—would Pam and her husband be willing to have their profile shown to the mother? They would. They met her in early September, and their son was born September 21. "We hadn't done a thing! We really thought we'd have a match and have two or three months to get ready," she says. The adoption was finalized in April 2010.

Costs and Support

Like fertility preservation and IVF, adoption can be costly. Unlike fertility preservation and IVF, adoption isn't covered by your health insurance. Once a child is legally in your custody—even before an adoption is finalized—your health insurance is required to cover their health care just as it would a child born to you, but that doesn't mean it has to pay for the adoption itself.

Costs of adoption vary widely. Some private domestic adoptions can be completed for less than $10,000, but that's rare. A 2009 survey done by *Adoptive Families* magazine found that over 50 percent of domestic newborn adoptions were completed with fees of less than $25,000, but 12 percent cost more than $30,000. A recent post to an adoption mailing list mentioned an agency seeking a family on the West Coast for twins soon to be born; fees were $45,000.[1]

International adoption is even more expensive because you pay all the same fees you usually pay in domestic adoption—agency fees for advertising and operations cost, legal fees, and so on—in addition to specific fees mandated by the country you're adopting from, as well as the costs of travel, sometimes multiple trips. Cost may be a big factor in terms of choosing a country—Russia, for example, can be particularly costly to adopt from given that it requires adoptive parents to take two separate trips. In *Adoptive Families'* 2009 survey, virtually everyone who adopted from Russia said their expenses had totaled more than $35,000. Nearly 70 percent of those adopting from Ethiopia, however, had costs totaling less than $25,000.[2]

Adopting from foster care is much less costly. In fact, in most cases, it ultimately costs parents nothing to adopt from foster care, and until you officially adopt your child, you will likely receive a monthly stipend from the state to cover some of their expenses. Their health care will also be paid for by Medicaid. If you adopt a child with special needs or a medically fragile child, there's additional support. Some states may even continue the support after the adoption is finalized. Many states have Subsidized Adoption Programs for special-needs children (this may merely mean that they are older, part of a sibling group that can't be separated, or from a minority group), which provide regular monthly support and Medicaid coverage until the adopted child turns eighteen or finishes high school.

If you're pursuing private domestic adoption or intercountry adoption, how do you go about affording it? There's no such thing as adoption insurance, and very few people have tens of thousands of dollars just sitting around waiting to be put to good use.

Tax Credit

If your adjusted gross income (AGI) is less than $122,000, you can receive a tax credit of $12,150 (as of 2009) for adoption. That means you can subtract up to $12,150 of documented adoption expenses (including travel) from your tax liability. You can split the credit into multiple years—for example, if you incur some agency expenses in 2010 and then more costs in 2011, when you finalize the adoption, you can take part of the credit on your 2010 tax bill and the rest in 2011. But if you're adopting internationally, you *cannot* take any part of the credit until the tax year that your adoption is finalized and your child becomes a U.S. citizen. You can find out more at www.irs.gov/taxtopics/tc607.html.

Employer Support

Many larger employers—and even some not-so-large ones—offer some kind of support to their employees who adopt. My husband's company, a financial services firm in New York, paid $5,000 toward the cost of our daughter's adoption. AstraZeneca, Bank of America, Capital One, Honeywell, KPMG, McGraw-Hill, MetLife, Microsoft, Patagonia, Warner Music Group, and several others have been praised by their employees for offering adoption assistance ranging from $5,000 to $10,000 per adoption.

Wheaton College of Illinois has a great policy—they provide equivalent benefits for adoptive families as if they were having children biologically. In terms of subsidies, that means they provide an approximation of the insurance costs for a normal, healthy delivery—about $10,000.

If your company hasn't caught on yet, you can make the case to them yourself that it's a great way to attract and retain excellent employees. Download the *Adoptive Families'* sample letter here: www.adoptivefamilies.com/articles.php?aid=1480.

Military Subsidies

The U.S. military provides up to $2,000 per child, or $5,000 per year, in support to military families who adopt, provided that they use a qualified adoption agency. These benefits aren't paid until the adoption is complete. You can find out more at www.childwelfare.gov/pubs/f_milita.cfm.

Grants and Loans

Many adoption agencies, and some private funds and charities, provide grants or loans to parents who adopt a waiting child or a child with special needs. You can find lists of these organizations at http://www.affordingadoption.com/grants.php. This organization has also just begun forming its own foundation that will offer adoption grants.

The National Adoption Foundation (www.nafadopt.org) uses a combination of corporate and private funds to offer grants, unsecured loans, and an "adoption credit card," open to all adoptive families, regardless of income and where you are adopting from. Grants range from $500 to $2,500.

Other Options

If you own your home, you might also consider a Home Equity Line of Credit (HELOC) to help finance adoption costs. The interest on the loan is tax-deductible, and you can usually write checks on the loan for just the amount you need. For example, if you're approved for a $20,000 HELOC, you can pay your individual bills using the loan rather than taking the whole amount out in one lump sum.

If you've definitely chosen adoption, you can probably skip the next chapter—on having a healthy pregnancy—and jump ahead to the following one on special parenting concerns after cancer. But if there's any chance that a postcancer pregnancy might be in the cards for you, don't miss chapter 6!

I'm Pregnant—Now What?

A Healthy Pregnancy After Cancer

THE DAY I FOUND OUT I was pregnant with my son, as soon as I stopped doing a goofy dance of joy in my bedroom, I thought, "Okay . . . so what do I do now?"

I hadn't really thought much past the getting pregnant part. Since that had seemed like such an insurmountable hurdle, all my focus had been on when and whether we would get pregnant—not what we'd do once I was, and whether or not being a cancer survivor would affect any of the big and little things involved with a pregnancy. Was I high risk? Would I have to have a C-section? Could I possibly see a midwife instead of an obstetrician? Would I be able to breast-feed after breast cancer? Would I have to see my oncologist more often? Oh crap—I hadn't even told my oncologist I was trying to get pregnant! What would she say?

To the list of a million questions every woman has about pregnancy, cancer survivors can add a litany of specialized concerns of their own. For many of us, the first question is "Is it safe?" In other words—is it going to make your cancer come back? For many cancer survivors, that's not an issue. Biologically speaking, nobody really expects that a pregnancy might lead to a recurrence of leukemia, thyroid cancer, or melanoma. But for women with breast cancer, who make up a fairly substantial percentage of cancer survivors still of reproductive age, the picture has long been a lot less clear. After all, breast cancer is, in many cases, fed by hormones such as estrogen and progesterone. And what happens during pregnancy? Your hormone levels go off the charts. Even if your tumor was ER/PR-negative (and therefore not fueled by the hormones estrogen and progesterone), a woman who's been through breast cancer could be forgiven for being just a little bit nervous about taking on a condition that is pretty much guaranteed to set off a lot of activity in the breasts.

Here's the good news: so far, there does not appear to be any scientific evidence that pregnancy causes breast cancer to recur. "That doesn't seem to make sense at first," says Dr. Chung. "The whole relationship between estrogen and breast cancer is so well established: estrogen leads to breast cell proliferation and an increased risk of recurrence. Pregnancy being a high-estrogen state, it was always thought to be a bad thing for women with breast cancer."

Despite that, a number of studies have looked at women who became pregnant after a breast cancer diagnosis. So far, none has found any increased risk of recurrence or negative effect on survival. "Over twenty studies have examined this, and the data are consistent. If you get pregnant after successful cancer treatment, there seems to be no increased risk of recurrence," says Dr. Oktay. "The number of studies and the total number of patients is very reassuring. Pregnancy involves a lot of hormones, not just estrogen, and we don't know how all of them interact."[1]

As mentioned in the introduction, there are even a couple of studies that have found a possible protective effect—that is, women who get pregnant after breast cancer have a *decreased* risk of recurrence. That makes some sense—after all, it's pretty well established that pregnancy helps to protect against breast cancer in the first place, so maybe it could protect against recurrence. On the other hand, that finding might also be explained by what scientists call the "healthy subject" bias—you probably wouldn't try to get pregnant after breast cancer if you weren't doing well and feeling good in the first place.

But it might also have to do with some of those other pregnancy factors that Dr. Oktay mentioned. In late 2009, researchers reported that alpha-fetoprotein (AFP), a protein produced during pregnancy, inhibits the growth of breast cancer cells. Human chorionic gonadotropin (HCG), another pregnancy protein, also appears to slow breast cancer growth.[2]

There are limits to the studies done so far about pregnancy after breast cancer. They're all *retrospective*, meaning they look back at information they already have to see if patterns emerge. Two studies are now ongoing—one at Memorial Sloan-Kettering in New York and one at the Dana-Farber Cancer Institute in Boston—that are *prospective*, meaning that they recruit patients and then follow them for a period of time to see if the women who do get pregnant have any different outcomes than those who don't. Those studies will be a lot more definitive than the information we now have, but their results won't be out for a while.

But what if you had ER/PR-positive cancer—cancer specifically fed by hormones? If you ask many oncologists, and many cancer survivors, they will say no way, no how, it's a bad idea to get pregnant after having had hormone-positive cancer. But experts who are familiar with the research say hormone receptor status isn't an issue. "Studies have looked at node-positive and node-negative disease, and some have even controlled for hormone receptor status," says Dr. Oktay. "It doesn't seem to make a difference."

That's true, says Anne Partridge, MD, a medical oncologist at the Dana-Farber Cancer Institute and a leading expert in breast cancer in young women. "One study even stacked the deck and looked at women with less favorable cancers—in terms of stage and grade—who got pregnant, and compared them to women who had not gotten pregnant and who had *more* favorable cancers," she says. "Even though you'd expect that it would make pregnancy after breast cancer look bad, what happened was that it appeared that there was no effect on survival at all. In fact, there were fewer recurrences in people who had pregnancies."[3]

There's one area that's still unstudied: women with BRCA mutations (genetic mutations that increase the risk of breast and other gynecological cancers). Dr. Oktay says that there hasn't been enough research on women with these genetic mutations to determine if postcancer pregnancy is risky for them. In some cases, it might be, not so much because it would increase the risk of recurrence but because it could delay recommended preventive options, like removing the ovaries in order to protect against ovarian cancer. But research hasn't looked at those questions yet.

Of course, you're not a piece of data from a study—you're an individual. Only you, with the advice of your doctor, can decide if it's a good idea for *you*, personally, to get pregnant after breast cancer, or any type of cancer.

"For example, if you have really high-risk breast cancer— twenty-one positive lymph nodes, and you're Her2-negative so you're not going to get Herceptin—you have a very high risk, no matter what treatments we give you, of hearing from the breast cancer again," says Partridge. "For a patient like that, your doctor may think it's too risky for you to get pregnant, not because it's likely to bring on a recurrence, but because they think you're at high risk of having a recurrence in any case."

Ultimately, it's your decision, not your doctor's. "I have a patient right now who has four kids. She has a BRCA mutation and is at high risk for recurrence. She has had a great response to chemo and surgery, but she needs to get her ovaries out because she's at high risk for ovarian cancer," says Partridge. "She says to me in midtreatment, 'I really want another child.' I'm going, 'What are you *talking* about?' But I'm her doctor, and all I can do is advise her. I can't decide for her."

Are You High Risk?

Once you've decided that pregnancy is safe for you—or safe enough, or important enough that you're willing to take some level of unknown risk—and you've overcome the hurdles in the way of getting pregnant, you may next wonder if your pregnancy itself is high risk, either for you or your baby.

All other things being equal, the answer is usually no. "To my knowledge, there's no particular reason that a cancer survivor is necessarily a high-risk OB patient," says Dr. Chung. "I've had several patients come to me after breast cancer therapy and say, 'I'm ready to get pregnant—how do I need to be monitored?' As far as I know, there are no guidelines or recommendations. You don't need to do mammograms or breast ultrasounds or exams every month. And the birth and perinatal outcomes of women with cancer don't appear to show any additional risk of problems." Your baby probably doesn't face any additional risks, either. Studies have found that the children of cancer survivors are no more likely to have birth defects or chromosomal anomalies than other children.[4]

All that said, there are some specific situations where you do need to be watchful, at least. The most important is heart trouble. Pregnancy puts a strain on the heart, and so do many types of chemotherapy. If you had impaired cardiac function after completing chemotherapy (generally measured as a lowered *ejection fraction*, the volume of blood your heart pumps out to the rest of the body with each beat), then you may be at increased risk for cardiac problems during pregnancy. Your doctor will probably watch you carefully for symptoms such as shortness of breath or excessive swelling of your legs; he or she may also want you to get an echocardiogram or other cardiac function tests regularly.

Another risk factor is age. Many women who become pregnant after cancer do so after thirty-five, just because of the delays in the family-planning timeline that cancer can throw into the works. And once you're over thirty-five, obstetricians consider you *AMA*— of advanced maternal age. (That's a less insulting term than the one they used to use: *elderly primigravida*. Seriously, *elderly?* You need a walker at thirty-seven?) AMA pregnancies are generally considered to be higher risk overall because women over thirty-five tend to have more complications: miscarriage, gestational diabetes, placenta previa, preeclampsia (dangerously high blood pressure and protein in the urine), and so on. But just being over thirty-five alone doesn't mean you will develop any of those conditions, so if they don't actually arise, you aren't particularly high risk.

Your best bet is probably to talk to your treating oncologist after you've become pregnant, and ask if he or she thinks you need to have your pregnancy managed by a high-risk obstetrician. If you had an early-stage cancer and responded well to treatment, in many cases, the answer will probably be no. In that case, you can pretty much seek out whatever childbirth professional you feel most comfortable with.

When I got pregnant with my son, I just assumed I'd need a high-risk obstetrician, being forty and a cancer survivor. But when I called my oncologist's office in early August, not long after the pregnancy was confirmed, she said, "Nope. Nothing to worry about. See you in December" (my next scheduled follow-up).

So I found myself a fantastic group of certified nurse-midwives who practice near my home and deliver at a nearby hospital with a Level III Neonatal Intensive Care Unit (NICU). When I first came in to meet with them, they didn't even blink when I told them about my cancer history. One of the owners of the practice told me that I was far from the first cancer survivor they'd cared for during pregnancy. (I ended up having a C-section with my son because he was stubbornly breech—butt first instead of head first—but that had nothing to do with the cancer. With my daughter Katia, I had a successful, uncomplicated vaginal birth after Cesarean, or VBAC, attended by my midwives in the hospital.)

In fact, licensed midwives might be a particularly good option for cancer survivors because of the personal nature of their care and how well they get to know their patients. What you *don't* want, says Dr. Partridge, is a large obstetrical practice that operates like an assembly line. "If someone is running a 'factory' with an extraordinarily busy practice, they may not have the time to listen to your complaint and see the nuances," she says. "Midwives may spend more time with you. They may say, 'This just doesn't fit.' But whoever you see, you have to know yourself. Talk to your doctor or midwife and make sure they're familiar with your history and potential complications. You want them to recognize that the signs and differential diagnosis of problems can be different for you than it might be in a patient who's never been treated for cancer."

Pregnancy and Your Medications

As discussed in chapter 1, one thing doctors will unequivocally advise you *not* to do is to become pregnant while taking certain long-term cancer medications like Tamoxifen or Herceptin, or during the first few months after you've stopped taking these drugs, until they're flushed out of your system. Tamoxifen has been associated with pregnancy anomalies in animal studies, and Herceptin may cause low amniotic fluid levels.[5] But sometimes you follow your doctor's advice and the unexpected happens anyway. What should you do if you find yourself pregnant while taking Tamoxifen or Herceptin?

Michelle Rommelfanger had to grapple with that tough question. The Sacramento mom, who was twenty-nine and caring for two-year-old twin boys when she was diagnosed with breast cancer in 2007, had been on Tamoxifen a little over a year and was using an IUD to prevent pregnancy when she went in for an exam. She mentioned to her doctor that her period was a week late. One pregnancy test later, Michelle was in shock.

"Oh my God," she says. "When I was diagnosed with cancer, it was the scariest thing that had ever happened to me. But I felt like I had more confidence in my doctors. When I found out I was pregnant, they had no clue what to do. My obstetrician told me to terminate; the perinatologist said I didn't have to. Then the genetics department said they didn't know what the Tamoxifen would do to the baby or if my cancer would have a higher risk of recurrence. I was an emotional wreck. I remember just sitting in the doctor's office crying."

Michelle stopped taking Tamoxifen immediately. She was almost six weeks pregnant. Doctors told her that she had a couple of weeks to make her decision: carry the pregnancy to term and risk the unknown, or terminate the pregnancy. "I did so much research and spoke with so many medical professionals and family members, and ultimately I just had to go with my gut," she says. "My husband and I thought that this baby had a reason to be here. By all rights, I wasn't supposed to get pregnant, but I did. I felt like it was meant to be. Since nobody could definitely tell me that it would be bad for my child, then I wasn't going to live in fear of problems with the baby or the cancer."

So she continued the pregnancy, and today, Mira Eliana is a happy, healthy, thriving baby whose big brothers dote on her. There are still worries—some of the concerns about Tamoxifen's long-term effects in pregnancy are that it might cause similar complications to the drug DES, a synthetic estrogen used in the mid-twentieth century that put the daughters of women taking the drug when they got pregnant at higher risk for certain gynecological cancers. "But so far, she's beautiful and healthy and everything looks fine," says Rommelfanger.

Jill Lenz, then forty-one, faced a similar scare when she became pregnant just weeks after completing treatment with the targeted breast cancer drug Herceptin in 2008. "My doctor told me I'd have the drug out of my system by March and it would be okay then to try and get pregnant," she says. "I made an appointment with fertility doctors the last week of February, just to get the ball rolling, and it turned out I was already pregnant—even though we'd been struggling with infertility before I got cancer, and we had been actively not trying!"

But the biggest concern with Herceptin and pregnancy is its effect on amniotic fluid levels, and Lenz's were just fine. "The pregnancy was rough: I had swollen feet, hemorrhoids, and horrid acid reflux," she says. "But I really felt like I was magic. After convincing myself that I was going to have to accept the fact that I wouldn't have a child, the experience of being pregnant made me younger again." Her son was born in November 2009.

Lenz is considering trying for one more child with the frozen embryos she was able to conceive prior to starting treatment—she only ended up with three, so she knows the odds might not be in her favor. "I really feel very lucky that it happened the way it did," she says. "I always wanted to have two kids, and I think siblings are really good for one another, but we'll see. I'm really happy with the way things are right now."

Drugs like Tamoxifen and Herceptin generally have a prescribed end date—usually five years for Tamoxifen and a year for Herceptin. Young women taking the leukemia drug Gleevec, however, don't have a definite end date. The medication is nothing less than a wonder drug for chronic myelogenous leukemia, completely turning the prognosis around—but it's not a cure. It puts the disease into remission. So as long as you're taking Gleevec, you're okay. If you stop, what happens? Does the CML come back? There's no clear-cut answer.

Erin Zammett Ruddy, who chronicled her experiences with CML in articles and a blog for *Glamour* as well as the book *My So-Called Normal Life*, made the difficult decision to temporarily stop taking Gleevec to become pregnant—not once, but twice. With her first son, she stopped taking the drug as soon as a sensitive early test confirmed pregnancy; she breast-fed for a month and then switched to formula so she could go back on Gleevec. While trying to get pregnant with her second child, her doctor felt more confident in her ability to remain in remission while off the drug, so he had her stop taking it as soon as she ovulated— and go back on if she got her period.

"This stopping and starting treatment was not ideal (my doctor's words: 'Is this what we recommend to patients? Heck no'), but given my previous success with getting pregnant fast and staying in remission, it was a pretty good option," Erin wrote for Parenting.com. "And it put the risk on me, not the baby, which is the way I prefer it. Fortunately I didn't have to do it for long. After the third cycle, I was pregnant." Her daughter, Nora, was born in January 2010.

Erin faced some criticism for her choice but maintains it was the right decision for her. Through her blog, she said, she has talked to several other young women who made the same choice, and although most of them experienced some form of relapse, they were able to have healthy babies and do well after going back on Gleevec.

Karla Vinson (name changed at her request) found out she had leukemia while pregnant with her second child, a daughter. Routine early pregnancy blood work came back with a startlingly high white count, and further testing ultimately revealed chronic myelogenous leukemia. At the time, Gleevec was relatively new on the scene. Some family members thought Karla should terminate the pregnancy and go on Gleevec immediately. But her oncologist, the husband of a close friend, called Brian Druker, the Oregon oncologist who developed the drug, and sought his expert advice. "They both felt that it would be okay to start the drug at thirty weeks," says Karla. "Since they've found that Gleevec causes developmental problems in lab rats, my oncologist felt that at thirty weeks, everything that needed to develop was pretty much developed. Dr. Druker agreed that that would be a safe time."

Karla went through a scary first two trimesters, watching her white count jump every time she had blood work done (at two-week intervals) and knowing she and her doctors could not do anything yet. At twenty-seven weeks, she went into preterm labor and was put on medication and bed rest at home. "At that point, my white count was 100,000, which was the point that everyone had said, 'Well, then we'd have to do something,'" Karla recalls. "Luckily, I wasn't very anemic, my spleen wasn't swollen, and my platelet levels were still good. My perinatologist wanted me to start Gleevec at twenty-seven weeks, because his feeling was if the mom's not healthy, the baby's not healthy. But because nothing else was out of whack too much, my oncologist felt we could wait a little bit."

Finally, at thirty weeks exactly, Karla's blood count had reached 149,000, and she started Gleevec. Because there are no tests to show what the drug does to an unborn child, Karla would have naturally preferred to wait until the baby was born—but she says that there was one positive note about starting the drug when she did. "The first couple of months, Gleevec makes you extremely sick, achy, and tired, because it's killing all those white cells," she says. "So I basically slept all day while my family took care of my son. And the achiness was horrible—Tylenol is the only pain reliever you can take while pregnant, but you can't take it while on Gleevec, because both drugs are metabolized by the same liver enzymes. It would have been very hard to have a new-born and feel like that."

Ultimately, she gave birth to her daughter at thirty-seven weeks of pregnancy, after being cleared to go off bed rest at thirty-six weeks. "By the time she was born, I had improved a lot. And just not having the strain of pregnancy on my body made me feel a lot better," Karla says. "She's a strong, athletic kid—we joke that all that medication built this bionic woman! And I'm still on Gleevec and still in full remission. My doctor hopes that after five years, I might be able to go off it entirely and live a normal life."

So Michelle Rommelfanger, Jill Lenz, and Karla Vinson all took cancer-related medications while pregnant—and all had happy endings, despite the previously mentioned lab and animal research that indicates a risk of birth defects or other health problems and despite the fact that little is known about how this might play out in humans. That doesn't mean, of course, that the same thing will happen to the next woman who unknowingly, or in a carefully thought-out plan, takes Tamoxifen, Herceptin, Gleevec, or another cancer drug during pregnancy. If you have to face the same decisions that these women faced, there's really no road map. But if there's something to be learned from these three women, it's the same thing that Anne Partridge tells her patients about when and if to get pregnant after breast cancer: you can get advice from your doctors and other people whose opinion matters to you, but ultimately, the choice is up to you. Only you know how much risk to yourself, and to a baby, you're ready to accept. Don't let anyone tell you that you "have to" terminate a much-wanted pregnancy because of early exposure to a drug with uncertain consequences for a developing fetus—but don't dismiss those concerns out of hand, either. Gather information, listen to the experts, and then listen to yourself.

Surgery Aftermath

If you've had surgery in the pelvic region, that *might* have an impact on your pregnancy. Because types of surgery, types of incision, and extent of surgery varies so much from patient to patient, it's hard to say whether a particular type of operation would make your pregnancy any riskier.

One surgery that is common in young breast cancer survivors who may later want to become pregnant is *breast reconstruction*, using tissue from the abdomen to re-create the missing breast tissue. TRAM (transverse rectus abdominis myocutaneous) flap surgery uses skin, tissue, and abdominal muscle; DIEP (deep inferior epigastric perforator) flap surgery uses skin, tissue, and fat, sparing the abdominal muscle. These surgeries don't directly affect your uterus, but they may leave less room (skin/muscle/tissue) for your belly to expand with a growing pregnancy.

It's considered safe to become pregnant after TRAM or DIEP flap surgery, although you may have some additional pregnancy-related challenges. Many women who've become pregnant after TRAM or DIEP flap have had no problems at all other than perhaps a slight feeling of tightness, and others have faced more significant issues such as herniations and confinement to a wheelchair during the last months of pregnancy.

Joseph Serletti, MD, chief of the Division of Plastic Surgery at the University of Pennsylvania, told Breastcancer.org in 2007 that he had had more than ten patients become pregnant and carry to term postreconstruction. None of them had any problems, he said, although most ended up delivering by C-section because of their prior abdominal surgery. Robert Allen, MD, who pioneered the DIEP flap procedure, agrees that DIEP patients can have normal pregnancies and deliveries.[6] Of course, anyone who's had significant surgery to their abdomen and pelvis—whether it's related to cancer or not—should talk to their doctor about possible pregnancy complications.

Screening During Pregnancy

Is it safe to undergo your usual cancer screenings and follow-up tests during pregnancy? Usually, yes, although it may not be necessary or useful.

For example, most breast cancer survivors undergo regular follow-up screening mammograms and/or breast MRIs, especially during the first five years after treatment. It may make you nervous, but small studies have found that mammography poses little to no harm to the fetus during pregnancy if a lead shield is placed on the belly to block any possible radiation scatter. Your doctor may suggest waiting until the second trimester, after most of the important development of fetal organs is complete, to get your mammogram. Or she may say that you can wait until after you deliver. That's because mammograms during pregnancy are notoriously inaccurate. Studies have found that mammograms detect significantly fewer breast cancers in pregnant women than in nonpregnant women.[7] When I got pregnant with my daughter, I called to change a mammogram appointment that was scheduled for what ended up being my fourth week of pregnancy. My oncologist said that, at five years posttreatment, I could just wait until I had the baby to reschedule the mammogram.

Breast-feeding can also make mammograms more difficult to read, as the breast tissue becomes very dense during lactation. Your doctor may want to wait to do your next screening mammogram until after you've weaned your baby. But if you're an extended breast-feeder and this will cause too much of a delay, you can help to get the clearest reading by nursing your baby immediately before the scan and emptying both breasts as much as possible. It is absolutely safe for breast-feeding mothers to have mammograms.

Even though pregnancy and breast-feeding can cause difficulties with reading mammograms, if you feel something suspicious in your breast during pregnancy or while nursing, as a cancer survivor (of any kind—even if your previous cancer wasn't in the breast), you should have it checked out. That may mean a mammogram, or a breast ultrasound, which is considered safe in pregnancy (after all, you'll probably go through a few ultrasounds to check out your baby's development).

What about X-rays, MRI scans, and PET scans? Most experts say that a single X-ray or MRI during pregnancy, especially after the first trimester, is unlikely to be harmful to a developing fetus. (In fact, a recent study found that MRI is a good tool to use in diagnosing placenta accreta, a pregnancy condition in which the placenta attaches too deeply into the uterus.[8]) But PET scans and CT scans are usually not recommended during pregnancy because they involve higher levels of radiation, even though no single use of an imaging tool (X-ray, MRI, PET, CT) has enough radiation to harm a fetus. Odds are you won't have any serious symptoms during your pregnancy that might call for a CT or PET scan, but if you do, your doctor will discuss with you the relative risks versus the importance of an accurate diagnosis. (With a cancer survivor, they might be a little more proactive about investigating something suspicious rather than just waiting watchfully.)

Beyond these questions, women who've had cancer should do pretty much all the same things for a healthy pregnancy that cancer-free women should do—that is, eat a balanced diet heavy on fruits and vegetables and low on processed foods; take prenatal vitamins daily (and for several months before trying to conceive); get regular exercise and plenty of sleep; and avoid smoking and alcohol. Heck, if your bout with cancer gave you the kick in the pants you needed to start eating better and working out more to improve your general health and, hopefully, cut your risk of recurrence, you might actually be in a *better* position to have a healthy pregnancy than an ordinary "healthy" woman who takes her cancer-free body for granted and doesn't actually pay that much attention to her health.

Breast-Feeding After Cancer

I was about six months pregnant with my son when I looked in the mirror while getting dressed one day and yelped something like, "Holy crap!" My left breast—the cancer-free one—had grown to the expected pregnancy-porn-star proportions. But the right breast, "cancer boob," had stayed pretty much the same size it had been before. Already a little bit smaller than Lefty because of the lumpectomy, it now was a dwarf by comparison—think 36B versus 38D.

This was a development I hadn't been expecting. I raced to my computer, and fifteen minutes later, had come up with the answer: breasts that have undergone radiation generally don't ever lactate again. In other words, if I wanted to breast-feed, I'd have to do it on one side alone. When I mentioned the prospect to a friend, she said, "Wow . . . that's gonna be one sore boob!"

For women who've had most types of cancer, breast-feeding after pregnancy isn't a big issue. You either do or don't, can or can't, just as you otherwise might have if you'd never had a cancer diagnosis. (Note: It is not considered safe to breast-feed *during* chemotherapy or radiation.)

But after breast cancer, breast-feeding is a whole different world. First, of course, if you've had a double mastectomy, you won't be able to breast-feed at all. There are milk banks around the country that can provide donor milk if it's very important to you to give your child this nutritional benefit. You can find out more from the Human Milk Banking Association of North

America at www.hmbana.org. But "donated" milk isn't free—it generally costs upwards of $2.00 per ounce. It may be possible to recruit a friend with a baby to pump some for you, but given how much time she'd be spending either nursing her own child or pumping for yours, she'd have to be a pretty good friend!

Even if you have one or both breasts left, breast-conserving surgery and radiation can damage the breast's ability to lactate. Your lumpectomy, although it may have spared most of your breast, might have damaged your milk ducts. As mentioned in chapter 1, if you are still planning surgery and want to preserve the prospect of nursing a child later, it's worth talking to your surgeon about whether or not he or she can make a surgical plan that will spare the milk ducts as much as possible.

External beam radiation doesn't linger in the treated breast—in other words, nursing a baby on a breast that previously had radiation doesn't pass along any aftereffects of the radiation to the baby. (As mentioned before, you can't breast-feed while actively getting radiation or chemotherapy.) But radiation does limit future milk production in the affected breast. In one study, only one of thirteen women who became pregnant after radiation to their breasts was able to produce milk on the irradiated side.[9]

When I had my son, other women who'd been pregnant after breast cancer recommended that I bring a breast pump to the hospital and pump on the "cancer side" right after I nursed him on the "good side," to stimulate milk production there without frustrating my newborn when he tried to nurse on a recalcitrant breast. I dutifully did so, but never got a single drop of colostrum or milk out of "cancer boob." After a few days, I decided not to waste my time and instead to focus my attention on making sure I could nurse well on the unaffected breast. But Pat Shelly, director of the Breastfeeding Center for Greater Washington in Washington, D.C., has seen radiated breasts successfully "primed" by a combination of pumping and hand expression in later pregnancy and the first few days after birth, so definitely give it a try. (Maybe I didn't start soon enough?)

Is it possible to nurse successfully on only one breast? Absolutely. It might not work for every individual, but it can be done. Think of it this way: some women breast-feed twins, which pretty much equates to one breast per baby. One woman who posts frequently on the Young Survival Coalition message boards calls the single breast on which she nursed her baby her "Power Boob."

Through a combination of luck (decent supply) and sheer German midwestern pigheadedness, I managed to nurse my son on one breast exclusively until he was seven and a half months old. It wasn't easy—especially at first. Adrian nursed about every two hours, and wanted to stay latched on for forty-five minutes at a stretch. I was exhausted. For the first couple of months, I alternated between loving breast-feeding and threatening to run out and buy out the formula aisle at Babies R Us. But then we got into a groove, and it became the most awesome thing I'd ever done.

Between seven and eight months, my voracious little guy got to be too much for me and I couldn't pump enough to keep up with his demands for three days a week at day care, so I supplemented with formula for day care until he was old enough to take cow's milk on those days. But when he was with me, he nursed— for a full two years.

Christina Demosthenous nursed her son for six months on one breast. "I was one of those women who was obsessed with breast-feeding," she says. "I didn't give him formula for four months—and he was a big kid, almost ten pounds! I don't think I moved from the chair or bed those first few months—he was nursing like every forty minutes."

Breast-feeding is fraught with emotion for many women. The "mommy wars" on many websites may start with reasonable discussions about the benefits of breast-feeding versus the challenges many women face, ranging from tongue-tie to babies who don't latch to inadequate supply to poor support—but they often devolve into "Formula is poison!" versus "Militant breast-feeders are Nazis!" arguments.

And when you're a breast cancer survivor trying to breast-feed, the whole thing gets even more emotional. After all, your breasts let you down once. They got cancer—or, at least, one of them did. The idea that they might not be able to do the very thing they were meant to do in the first place—nourish a baby—can make you even angrier at your body. For me, being able to breast-feed my son for so long was a huge deal, because along with the pregnancy itself, it felt like a big "in your face" to cancer. Not only did you not kill me, but you didn't take away my ability to be a mother and you couldn't even stop me from breast-feeding. I win.

But sometimes we *don't* win that particular battle. Sometimes women just don't have enough supply. (There are plenty of women with *two* functioning breasts who have supply issues, so when you're working with half the troops, there's all the more chance of difficulty.) Sometimes you might have to go back to work and pumping on one breast all the time is too difficult. Or you might get mastitis on that single breast, or a nipple that cracks and bleeds endlessly because it never gets a break.

Courtney Bugler struggled with supply issues from the beginning. "My son was nine pounds at birth, and I could just never get my one breast to make enough," she says. "He was eating six ounces a feeding by two weeks! We had to supplement from the beginning. After a few weeks, my husband looked at me sitting there pumping all the time, and he said, look, the last thing you need is to have more issues with what your breasts are and are not doing to you."

"But it's better for him!" Courtney protested.

"You happier is better," her husband responded.

"Within a day and a half of making the choice to stop, I was a whole new person," she says.

Jill Lenz had the same experience. "I didn't produce that much on my good side—I could barely make three ounces," she says. "Before getting pregnant and having a child, I wanted to breast-feed because it was the right thing to do. But by the time I had to wean, I was crying about it because of the bonding we'd had."

So if breast-feeding after breast cancer can be such a challenge and so stressful, why try to do it at all? Well, you probably already know about the body of research indicating that breast-feeding—even for a few weeks—has great nutritional and immunological benefits for the baby. (Even just getting the early milk, the colostrum, is like liquid gold for your child.) Breast-feeding appears to help protect babies from diarrhea, gastrointestinal problems, respiratory infections, ear infections, and allergies. It may even protect your child from leukemia and diabetes later in life. And as many women will tell you, the bonding experience while nursing your baby is amazing—perhaps all the more so when you may have recently had a very hate-love relationship with your breasts.

But for a breast cancer survivor, another very important factor about breast-feeding is its health benefits for *you*. It's been strongly established that breast-feeding helps to protect against all forms of breast cancer—hormone-positive or hormone-negative. In fact, a 2009 study found that breast-feeding reduced the risk of developing breast cancer for women with a family history of the disease by 59 percent![10] Most studies suggest that the longer you breast-feed, the greater its protection. Now, it's unknown if this protective effect also applies to breast cancer *recurrence*, because most studies haven't tried to tease that out. But it certainly would make sense that the protective effect would still apply when it comes to cancer recurrence, and there's absolutely no evidence that breast-feeding is in any way risky for a breast cancer survivor.

So for all of those reasons, many of us who've survived breast cancer want to give breast-feeding the best chance we can. How can you maximize your chances of successfully breast-feeding on one breast? Pat Shelly, who has worked with at least twenty women who've breast-fed after breast cancer, has some tips:

1. **Plan ahead.** Start getting ready to breast-feed while you're still pregnant. As soon as you see a bit of milk coming from the "good" breast during pregnancy, start trying to hand-express milk from the other breast, and periodically sit down with the pump. "It stimulates growth in areas that have been compromised, and builds your confidence," she says.

2. **Seek out support**—*informed* support. My otherwise absolutely wonderful and rather crunchy obstetrician informed me in the hospital that I should only nurse ten minutes "on each side" or I'd become engorged. (She kept forgetting I only had one "side.") Luckily, I'd read enough to know that wasn't true and kept on nursing my baby as long as he wanted. Use the kellymom.com directory at www.kellymom.com/lcdirectory/index.html to find a lactation consultant near you; you can also ask your obstetrician, pediatrician, and friends who've breast-fed. Call a few lactation consultants before you give birth to see whom you're most comfortable with, and ask if they've ever worked with breast cancer survivors before. You can also attend lactation classes at the hospital where you'll deliver. The support you get should also come from your family and friends. Talk to your husband and other family members ahead of time about how important

breast-feeding is to you, and tell them that you will need their encouragement to keep going, not comments like, "You can always quit." You *know* you can quit. You'll need to hear that you're doing great.

3. **Plan on intense breast-feeding during the first month or so.** Breast-feeding during the first couple of months isn't easy even for women with two functioning breasts. Set yourself up with *lots* of support for the early weeks and expect that during that time, you'll basically be a breast with baby attached. Breast-feeding is a demand and supply issue—the more you nurse, the more milk you make, especially early on. Don't give yourself a schedule: nurse your baby as often and as long as he or she wants. And practice *kangaroo care* between feedings—that means lots of skin-to-skin contact. "Each minute that goes by with the baby close to your chest, your body is seeping with oxytocin hormones that can help milk come in faster," Shelly says.

4. **Care for your overworked breast.** Don't wait until after your nipple starts getting sore, peeling, or cracked to apply nipple cream like Lansinoh—do it daily from the get-go. (Don't, however, follow the old wives' tale that advises rubbing the nipple with a rough washcloth to "toughen it up." That will make them even more tender when you start nursing.) Actually, I ended up replacing my lanolin cream with a cheaper alternative—breastmilk. I had read about breastmilk's natural healing properties, so I tried rubbing a little expressed milk on the nipple a couple of times a day and letting it air-dry before putting my top back on— never once had a cracked or bleeding nipple. You can even start doing this before the baby is born, late in pregnancy when your colostrum starts to come in.

5. **Buy different equipment.** The standard nursing bras
    don't work too well for us one-boobed nursers. One cup
    is full to overflowing and the other is half-empty and
    drooping. To address this problem, either get fitted for a
    "cutlet"—a small bra implant—at your cancer center or
    a lingerie shop, or skip the nursing bra entirely and go
    with a nursing tank instead. The tank has a more uniform
    effect, so the smaller side isn't as floppy as with a half-
    empty bra cup. It's still noticeably smaller, though, so
    if you have an issue with looking a little lopsided, go
    with the cutlet. I went with the tanks, which are oh-
    so-comfortable and making nursing in public super-easy.
    But I still wound up blushing a bit, like when a clerk at
    Target told me she knew my son was breast-fed because,
    "You look really engorged on that side!" Once I picked
    my chin up off the floor, I gently informed her about the
    whole cancer thing.

6. **Handle supplementation carefully.** If you have to supple-
    ment early on due to low supply, do it in a way that doesn't
    encourage your baby to prefer a bottle. "Some babies can
    easily be 'ambidextrous,' while others can have a strong
    bottle preference," says Shelly. "Hold the bottle horizon-
    tally, not vertically, so the baby has to pull at the nipple
    rather than having milk drip into [his or her] mouth. That
    makes [the baby] less likely to prefer the bottle because
    getting milk from it is easier." While you're feeding your
    baby a pumped bottle, be sure to give lots of skin-on-skin
    time so that the baby learns to associate skin-to-skin con-
    tact (as with nursing) with a full tummy. And don't forget
    to pump right around the time of any bottle feedings to
    encourage milk supply.

Once you've successfully made the journey to parenthood—whatever your path—it doesn't mean that cancer stops being relevant. Those of us who've faced cancer have a much more intimate relationship with our mortality, at a much younger age, than people who haven't. And that can affect how we think about parenting, and our plans, hopes, and fears for our children. As we cuddle our kids, the "what ifs" can be hard to ignore. In the next chapter, we'll talk about how to put cancer in perspective when you're a parent.

CHAPTER 7

What's Cancer, Mom?

Fears and Concerns About Parenting After Cancer

AS I'M WRITING THIS CHAPTER, it's been more than six years since I first found the lump in my right breast. I've passed the fabled five-year survivor mark, and "graduated" to the survivorship program at Sloan-Kettering—fewer follow-up visits, and only with the nurse practitioner instead of the oncologist unless something seems hinky.

Cancer's on my mind a lot now because I'm writing this book, but most of the time I can go for days or weeks without even thinking about having had cancer. It's just a chunk of my biography— I grew up in Nebraska, I love Ethiopian food and figure skating, I drive a minivan, my favorite writer is Robertson Davies, and I had breast cancer.

But then . . . the land mines come along and trip me up, reminding me that I'm not like all the other moms. Like when I recently started calling insurance companies, figuring that as a five-year survivor I might be able to get life insurance again. When I was diagnosed, I wasn't a mom. No one was depending on me for the things they needed to live. Life insurance wasn't even on my radar screen. Now, with three kids, and with my income accounting for about half of our family's support, life insurance has suddenly gotten a lot more important.

But when I started making calls, I found out that my cancer seems a lot more immediate to the insurance companies than it does to me. Five years and the words *pathological complete response* doesn't mean much to them. If I want to get life insurance that doesn't cost a giant chunk of our monthly budget, I have to be at least *seven* years out from treatment. One company wouldn't even talk to me until I was *ten* years out.

That'll bring you up short. Yeah, life insurance companies are just trying to minimize their risk, so it makes sense—but it's still a stark reminder that you're not like everybody else. Despite how good you feel, the people who do the math say you might not be here next year.

That's a hard reality for any cancer survivor to face. But when you're a cancer survivor with young children—or trying to *have* young children—it's not just you, your husband, or your grown kids that you're scared for. It's that baby or that two-year-old or that five-year-old, who still needs you for *everything*. Or who will, even if he or she isn't here yet.

How do you deal with that burden? There's the not-so-abstract ethical question of "Is it right to bring a child into my world and promise to take care of them, when I'm not entirely sure I'll be here for their first day of kindergarten?" And then, once you've grappled with that, there are also the questions about how much, when, and if you talk to your kids about having had cancer in the first place.

For Jilda Nettleton, the fears of what might happen if the cancer comes back aren't abstract at all; hers already has. Her daughters, Aileen and Reanne, were three and nine months when Jilda's DCIS (ductal carcinoma in situ—limited to the ducts and not yet spread to the rest of the breast tissue) breast cancer recurred in 2008. She knows that the recurrence might well have happened because she chose to wait a year and a half after treatment to go on Tamoxifen so that she could get pregnant and give birth to Aileen and then went back off Tamoxifen after a year to have Reanne.

"I know that with DCIS the prognosis is so much better," Jilda says. "But you still think, am I going to be the person who goes from DCIS to stage IV? I know people [to] whom that's happened. . . . I don't think about it every day, but there are times when it's there in the back of my head. What if something else happens, and I do get very unlucky and I don't get to see my kids grow up? In my support group, one woman died who had kids the same age as mine, and it was so hard to see that and think of that. But I have to just make the most of every day and be sure that I'm doing the best that I can to take care of myself."

Jilda says she's very open with her daughters about medical issues—even at their young ages. "I still have to go to a lot of doctor's appointments and I don't try to hide anything. My kids know the word cancer," she says. "My four-year-old asks a lot of questions, and I do my best to answer honestly. They are familiar with the fact that bad things happen—I don't try to shield them from that."

I take the same approach Jilda does. One night, my then four-year-old daughter looked at me in the bathtub and asked why "That one looks different from that one," pointing at my breasts. I explained that before she was born, Mommy had a sickness called cancer, and it made a lump that the doctors had to take out to make me well. They made a cut in my breast and took it out, and then sewed me up and also gave me medicine to make me better. We talked a lot about where the scar was and if it hurt. She never asked if I was sick enough to die . . . but I know that question will come up. And I'll have to tell her at least some of the truth (because if I lie to her, how will she ever trust me when she finds out?). "Sometimes people *do* die of cancer, but Mommy had very good doctors and they don't think my cancer is ever going to come back." Will that be enough to reassure her? I don't know. After all, it doesn't always totally reassure *me*.

Terri Turner, who both adopted and had a biological child after cancer, is particularly aware of her responsibility to the daughter she adopted. "There's a grave responsibility to adopting a child," she says. "The angst for me has been thinking about helping her deal with such a loss from her birth, and on top of that also worrying that I might die early—that she might lose *two* mothers. That's the fear that I have a problem with avoiding or hiding from. I just get apoplectic and panic every so often, like every time there's a cancer scare, and I've had a few since we brought her home."

Facing the prospect of parenting with cancer is an increasingly common scenario, according to Paula Rauch, MD, a child psychiatrist who directs the Parenting at a Challenging Time (PACT) program at Massachusetts General Hospital. "A pretty high percentage of the people still in treatment for cancer have children at home," she says. "And because the statistics on childhood cancer survivorship are so good, there's now a whole new population of grown-ups who survived pediatric cancer and are becoming parents. They're not in treatment, we don't see them at the clinic, but they're out there."[1]

Choosing to become a parent is always, in some way, a leap of faith. When you have a cancer history and fear what that might mean for your children, it's even more of a leap—and one that's not subject to logical analysis, Rauch says. "This is such a profound issue; it's not something for which you can get out a risks and benefits sheet and list the pros and cons. Like most difficult emotional things, people have a gut sense of what they want to do. In the sixteen years I've worked in our clinic, I've never met a parent who said they were undecided about having children." That said, if you're having trouble deciding whether having children is right for you, it can help you to talk to other people who've also faced the same dilemma. The message boards run by the Young Survival Coalition are a great place to connect with other survivors who've had kids or are thinking about it (there are boards for fertility, pregnancy, and parenting), as is the adoption-after-cancer Yahoo! Mailing list. For more on both, see Resources.

Rauch reminds all the parents she works with that nobody knows what their future holds. "In the course of working with patients who have a poor prognosis, it hasn't been uncommon that they've had any number of people in their circle of family and friends die unexpectedly," she says. "We all live with risk. Some of us are just more acutely aware of it than others."

As cancer survivors, we can take advantage of that awareness—no matter how painful it might be—to build stronger connections with our children, just as Jilda Nettleton describes. Here are some of Rauch's tips:

- Encourage your children to ask questions. "Set an atmosphere in the family that questions and curiosity are invited in," she says. "And when they do ask, make sure you understand what it is they're really wondering about. Try to tease out 'the question behind the question.'"

- Don't sweep problems under the rug or pretend upsetting things didn't happen. Make it a family value to talk about the difficult stuff.

- Build a circle of other caring adults who support your kids as well and are available to spend time with them and answer questions.

- Recognize that confidence comes from the ability to bear age-appropriate frustrations and disappointments. "Don't bubble wrap kids or prevent them from having knocks, bruises, physical and emotional bumps," Rauch says. "Give them the confidence that they can manage so they become hardy over time."

These kinds of coping techniques and support systems will strengthen your child no matter what—whether or not you experience a recurrence of your cancer. But in the event they do lose you, remember that the power of your love isn't measured in years. "Well-loved parents exist within their children long after they're gone," says Rauch. "The best gift a parent gives a child is a solid sense that they've been loved. It would be wonderful for everybody to have their parents forever, but kids often have very powerful feelings of being loved by and supported by a parent who has died. Sometimes kids tell me that they feel their parents' goodwill present with them and have a sense of courage: if they've faced this loss, how hard could the SATs be?"

As cancer survivors, we probably all have a more visceral sense of the shortness of days, and the preciousness of time, than people who've never faced a life-threatening illness. When it comes to our children, what should we do with that? Make memories and make them concrete, Rauch says. "When we've spoken with adults who lost their parents earlier in life and asked them if they had a letter or photo album, what they'd want it to say, they've said that they want to know what their parents saw in them that was special and what their parents' favorite memories were with them."

So obsess about those photo albums and scrapbooks even more than the average parent. Don't just stick pictures in the albums—annotate them, and write more than just "Jane at the lake, 2010." Instead, write something like, "Jane about to jump off the dock for the first time at Lake Wannasink, June 2010. I loved watching her stand with her toes poking off the boards, teetering on the edge, a little scared and a little excited, with that fierce, determined expression on her face."

Rauch suggests making a personal memory book for each child so that they can open it and follow the story of their life with you whenever they want. "Things that are highly emotional are harder if they fly in under your radar screen, so being able to look at these books when they want, in their own time, is good," she says.

Making books like this is easy now that there are online services like Shutterfly that can create professional-looking, beautiful bound volumes with your pictures and notes. Rauch knew one mom who'd created a "year in review" book for her family every year at Christmas, featuring fun family photos and all the things that were special that they'd done that year. "Those books became extra valuable when she became ill," Rauch says.

Another woman I know, who hasn't ever faced a serious illness, came up with an amazing tradition when her daughter was a baby that she still carries on now that the little girl is seven. Every week, she writes her daughter a "love letter," talking about all the fun things they did that week, what her daughter is learning and doing, and how special she is to her mom. Now, weekly might seem a little exhausting—but even doing that once a month, or once a year, will be a treasure for your child someday. All the more so if something happens to you—but it will be special to them even if it doesn't.

Take more pictures. Take more videos. Make more scrapbooks. And make sure they all tell the story of you. Don't forget to include *yourself*—parents are often the ones taking the pictures and the videos, and they inevitably become a compilation of the kids' exploits. Occasionally, turn the camera or the video recorder or the pen on yourself and record who *you* are, right now, so your kids won't forget. I didn't lose my mom young—she passed away in 2008, when she was seventy-four and I was forty-one—but I still wish she'd done more of that in her lifetime. She was an inveterate recorder of family stories—everyone's, that is, but hers.

Here are some other preparations you can make for your child in case "it" comes back:

1. **Establish rituals.** "Evidence suggests that rituals help people at difficult times. Even things as simple as Friday night 'breakfast for dinner' or Monday night pizza, these familiar things can reassure children," Rauch says.

2. **Make practical plans.** Many parents put off decisions about wills and guardianship, which is never a good idea, but even worse if you have any reason to be concerned about one parent's health. "Think very seriously about your guardianship decisions," Rauch advises. "If your child's potential guardians live somewhere else, or if your spouse might relocate if something happens to you, look for opportunities to make those places more familiar, like sending [your child] to summer camp in the area."

3. **Write a letter to your child explaining why you made the decisions you made about your life, your health, and having children.** "Sometimes something can happen very quickly, and you lose the ability to have that conversation," says Rauch. "Anticipating the questions your child might ask can be helpful. We see a lot of families in which the siblings were conceived in different ways—maybe one was adopted, one was biological, or one was conceived with a donor egg. Talk about the way in which everybody is loved equally and what went into the decision process."

Rauch's final rule: "When it comes to things that can be emotionally challenging, don't leave the story up to mystery."

Worth It All

Emotionally challenging. That's a good way to describe having children after cancer. Even at its "easiest," parenting can turn you inside out. But when you're building a family and caring for children in the shadow of cancer, there's always one more suitcase to tote with your emotional baggage.

But—and here, I don't want to sound like those sunny, perky, "cancer is a gift" sloganeers, but this is true—having had cancer also adds immeasurably to the rewards of having a child. Building a family is an undeniable expression of faith in the future. It's sending a part of yourself out into a time when you'll no longer be here. And it's trusting that you *will* be here long enough to instill the lessons, values, and love that your children need. Having and raising children, however you get there, is the ultimate declaration of victory over cancer. Cancer didn't win. It couldn't take this away.

So if you are committed to having a family, to loving a child, after cancer, then don't let chemotherapy, or low sperm counts, or a recalcitrant adoption agency, or a pile of paperwork the size of Mount Everest stop you. There's a path for you somewhere. Find it, make it, or beat it into submission. Because every parent in this book will tell you: the journey was hard, usually expensive, sometimes discouraging, and often exhausting, but it was always, *always* worth it.

Resources

THERE ARE SOME OUTSTANDING organizations, books, websites, and other resources out there for anyone coping with cancer in their reproductive years and thinking about their options for having a family afterward.

Organizations

Cancer and Fertility/Young People with Cancer

Fertile Hope/Livestrong

Fertile Hope is a national nonprofit organization that provides information about reproductive options for cancer survivors. They've been in the vanguard of the cancer and fertility movement for years. Their website, www.fertilehope.org, includes flowcharts of your fertility preservation and family-building options, risk calculators to help you determine how likely your treatment regimen is to damage your fertility, and information on financial support. In 2009, Fertile Hope was acquired by Lance Armstrong's Livestrong initiative, part of the Lance Armstrong Foundation. Their Sharing Hope initiative, providing financial assistance for fertility preservation and treatment for cancer survivors, is now part of Livestrong's Survivorcare program; you can find out more by calling 866-965-7205 or online at www .livestrong.org/survivorcare. Livestrong itself also has an extraordinary amount of resources for cancer survivors, especially younger people coping with cancer and its aftermath. Check out the main livestrong.org site.

The Oncofertility Consortium

A national research and patient support initiative focused on fertility and childbearing after cancer, the Oncofertility Consortium is housed at the Northwestern University Feinberg School of Medicine in Chicago. When you call their national fertility hotline, you'll be connected with an expert in cancer and fertility who can answer all your questions about treatment, fertility, fertility preservation options, cost, and other issues. They can also refer you to one of about two dozen Consortium members or other fertility preservation programs near you. Contact them at www.oncofertility.northwestern.edu, www.myoncofertility.org (their outstanding patient education website), or on the fertility hotline at 866-708-3378.

Young Survival Coalition (YSC)

YSC is the leading organization focused on the unique issues of young women with breast cancer—at last count, more than 250,000 women under the age of forty in the United States are currently diagnosed with or survivors of breast cancer, and approximately 10,000 more are diagnosed each year. YSC has an outstanding meeting every February for young survivors, and their online bulletin boards are a very active source of support—including one board about fertility issues and another board about pregnancy after breast cancer. Contact them at www.youngsurvival.org, info@youngsurvival.org, or 877-YSC-1011 (toll free).

Facing Our Risk of Cancer Empowered (FORCE)

FORCE is a support organization for women at high risk of breast and ovarian cancer due to family history and hereditary genetic mutations. FORCE hosts an annual conference for survivors and "previvors," operates a helpline and online message boards and chat rooms, and offers information on issues like finding specialists, getting financial support, and handling insurance issues. Contact them at www.facingourrisk.org, info@facingourrisk.org, or 866-288-RISK (toll free).

I'm Too Young for This! Cancer Foundation (i[2]y)

Focusing solely on the needs of young cancer survivors, i[2]y has a don't-miss radio show, *The Stupid Cancer Show*, as well as local chapters, happy hours, specialized support channels, and plenty of activism. Check them out at www.i2y.com.

General Fertility

RESOLVE: The National Infertility Association

RESOLVE offers support and education to women and men dealing with infertility of all kinds—including cancer-related infertility. They have educational videos about fertility options, links to support groups, and information about fertility treatment financing programs. Their website also offers contact information for fertility specialists, attorneys, and adoption agencies in your area (just note that while these professionals are members of RESOLVE, that doesn't mean the organization specifically endorses them). Contact them at www.resolve.org or 703-556-7172.

Society for Assisted Reproductive Technology (SART)

SART represents fertility and assisted reproduction specialists in the United States. If your fertility specialist is a SART member, this is a good thing. Their website offers step-by-step detailed guides through all aspects of the assisted reproduction process.

They also have an excellent "find a clinic" search tool that lets you compare fertility clinics' success rates in detail. For example, you can see how successful each clinic is with women in your age group using fresh or frozen eggs, a woman's own or donor eggs, and how many retrievals result in live births. Check out their website at www.sart.org.

American Society for Reproductive Medicine (ASRM)

ASRM is an education, standard-setting, and advocacy organization for fertility professionals. Like SART, they offer lots of patient education materials about infertility and the fertility treatment process, including a guide to state laws governing infertility insurance and guidelines on selecting an ART program. ASRM membership is also something to look for in your fertility professional; their website can connect you with ASRM members and other reproductive professionals. Contact them at www.asrm.org.

International Premature Ovarian Failure Association

This group is for any woman who has had premature ovarian failure—that means the loss of ovarian function before age forty—due to any cause, including cancer-related causes. They have an outstanding FAQ (frequently asked questions), referrals to local support groups, an email discussion list and message board, and a "Dr. Answer Line." Contact them at www.pofsupport.org or 703-913-4787.

The International Council on Infertility Information Dissemination, Inc. (INCIID)

INCIID (pronounced "inside") is a nonprofit organization providing information and support about all options for family building, including ART and adoption. Their discussion forums are moderated by experts in their fields, which is pretty cool. They also have a national "IVF Scholarship Program" called "From INCIID the Heart," which provides assistance with ART for families in financial need who don't have insurance coverage. It's not a grant program—"scholarship" recipients, who must be donating members of INCIID (at least $55 a year), get services donated by contributing doctors and facilities. Find out more at www.inciid.org or INCIIDinfo@inciid.org.

OPTS (the Organization of Parents Through Surrogacy)
OPTS is a national support network for parents who have built their families through surrogacy, are trying to, or are just thinking about it. They offer free online classifieds, professional listings, and lots of very informative background articles. They also have a popular email listserv that you can join by emailing bzager@msn.com. For more information, look them up online at www.opts.com or call 847-782-0224.

Adoption and Fostering

Evan B. Donaldson Adoption Institute
The Institute focuses on improving adoption access, making the process more equitable for everyone involved in adoption, and improving the ethics of adoption. From detailed research reports on topics ranging from transracial adoption and prenatal substance abuse and adoption, to educational webinars on topics like parenting children from "hard places," the Donaldson Institute has a wealth of information for everyone involved in adoption, including prospective adoptive parents. Whether you're considering adopting domestically, internationally, or through foster care, there's something here for you. Dedicate at least a couple of hours to reading the wealth of material on their website at www.adoptioninstitute.org; you can also contact them at 212-925-4089.

Adoption Learning Partners (ALP)

A great resource for preparing to become an adoptive family, ALP offers a variety of online educational resources for adoptive parents and prospective adoptive parents, on everything from creating an adoption profile that "works" to going from being a foster family to a forever family. Many of their courses may help you meet requirements from your adoption agency or state that are part of passing a home study. (The organization was founded in 2002 by respected Illinois adoption agency The Cradle.) Learn more at www.adoptionlearningpartners.org or by calling 800-566-3995.

National Resource Center for Recruitment and Retention of Foster and Adoptive Parents at AdoptUsKids

A collaborative venture of the Children's Bureau, Administration for Children and Families, and the Department of Health and Human Services, AdoptUsKids recruits foster and adoptive families and connects them with waiting children throughout the country. They also have state-by-state information on foster parent requirements, training, and how to contact local agencies. Learn more at www.adoptuskids.org.

Foster Care and Adoptive Community (FCAC)

FCAC offers 132 courses that can help you get certified to become a foster parent; they're also licensed in more than a dozen states to provide continuing education credit for social workers. In addition, they offer message boards, email listservs, and a host of enlightening articles. Find them online at www.fosterparents.com.

Dave Thomas Foundation for Adoption

This national nonprofit that promotes adoption from foster care publishes the very helpful guide, *A Child Is Waiting: A Step-by-Step Guide to Adoption.* They can also help you make the case for adoption benefits to your employer with their employee toolkits, and can help you educate yourself, your friends, and family, providing other background materials, including educational videos. Find out more at www.davethomasfoundation.org.

National Foster Parent Association (NFPA)

NFPA's tools for potential foster parents include extensive state-by-state resources, a complete tax guide, and local chapters that can provide support. They're online at www.nfpainc.org.

Books

Cancer and Fertility/Young People with Cancer

100 Questions and Answers About Cancer and Fertility, by Kutluk Oktay, MD, Lindsay Nohr Beck, and Joyce Dillon Reinecke, JD (Jones and Bartlett Publishers, 2008). This Fertile Hope publication provides practical, straightforward answers to questions about cancer and fertility.

Crazy Sexy Cancer Tips, by Kris Carr and Sheryl Crow (skirt!, 2007). It's been called the first "girlfriend's guide to living with cancer." Author Kris Carr calls herself a "cancer babe," and her hip, no-holds-barred, irreverent attitude to dealing with cancer and its aftermath are just what a lot of us need.

Everything Changes: The Insider's Guide to Cancer in Your 20s and 30s, by Kairol Rosenthal (Wiley, 2009). Let's face it, cancer when you're twenty-five and dating isn't the same as cancer when you're sixty and hugging grandchildren. Rosenthal, diagnosed with thyroid cancer at twenty-seven, interviewed other young survivors across the country for this guidebook/confessional mash-up.

Beauty Pearls for Chemo Girls, by Marybeth Maida and Debbie Kiederer (Citadel, 2009). Is it shallow to have a book of makeup and styling tips for women coping with cancer? Not at all! We deserve—hell, we *need*—to feel gorgeous and stylish too, even when we don't have eyelashes. And while you're probably not going to be trying to conceive a baby *during* treatment (at least, we hope you're not), it can't hurt to do your best to feel desirable and sexy throughout the process.

Let's Talk About It: Inspiring Stories from Young Adult Cancer Survivors, by Darren Neuberger (Authority Publishing, 2010). This is an awesome collection of real-world stories. You'll find someone you can relate to here.

General Fertility

Taking Charge of Your Fertility, by Toni Wechsler (Harper Paperbacks, 10th edition, 2006). Known as "TCOYF" among devotees, this book is the Bible of fertility awareness—that is, learning your own cycle and fertility signs. You may think you're having fertility problems because you "baby dance" every month dutifully around the middle of your cycle—but guess what? Maybe you ovulate on day 22, not day 14! Figure out when it's best to try to conceive, when you're at risk of miscarriage, and how your hormones and menstrual cycle work. This is a must-have.

What to Do When You Can't Get Pregnant: The Complete Guide to All the Technologies for Couples Facing Fertility Problems, by Daniel Potter, MD, and Jennifer Hanin (Da Capo Press, 2005). The book in your hands just scratches the surface of what assisted reproduction is all about; Potter and Hanin's book is your total guide to the medical, technological, and emotional labyrinth of fertility treatments.

Budgeting for Infertility: How to Bring Home a Baby Without Breaking the Bank, by Evelina Weidman Sterling and Angie Best-Boss (Fireside, 2009). All the reproductive technology in the world won't do you much good if you can't afford it, especially if your bank account has already been ravaged by bills for your cancer treatment. Recommended by the guru of fertility, Toni Weschler, this book is practical and thorough.

Making a Baby: Everything You Need to Know, by Debra Fulghum Bruce and Samuel Thatcher, MD (Ballantine Books, revised edition, 2010). This is a comprehensive resource covering everything from threats to your fertility and pregnancy at "midlife" to natural fertility solutions and assisted reproduction.

Adoption and Fostering

The Adoption Guide (*Adoptive Families* magazine, 2010). Published by *Adoptive Families* magazine, one of the most respected publications in the adoption world, this is a thorough and authoritative guide to all aspects of the adoption process—domestic, international, and foster. It covers how to get started, how to choose an agency or attorney, cost information, and "been-there, done-that" advice from adoptive parents about transitions for older children being adopted and managing an open adoption relationship. This book must be on your shelf if you're considering adoption. It's available in both a digital and print edition, with tons of online excerpts, at www.adoptionguide.com.

You Can Adopt: An Adoptive Families Guide, by Susan Caughman and Isolde Motley (Ballantine Books, 2009). Another awesome resource from the *Adoptive Families* professionals, combining guidelines and facts with powerful real-life stories, this book is comprehensive and honest.

The Complete Book of International Adoption: A Step by Step Guide to Finding Your Child, by Dawn Davenport (Broadway, 2006). Davenport, an attorney, international adoptive mom, and frequent writer on adoption topics, covers all the details of international adoption here. She presents a clear-eyed picture of the realities of adopting from another country—the joys and rewards as well as the responsibilities and challenges (like developmental delays and attachment issues). If you want to go into international adoption with your eyes open, read this book.

Success as a Foster Parent: Everything You Need to Know About Foster Care, by the National Foster Parent Association and Rachel Greene Baldino (Alpha, 2009). A clear, step-by-step guide to becoming a foster parent, with detailed information about what it entails, how to research agencies, the challenges involved, and how to deal with schools, physicians, vacations, and myriad other factors.

Practical Tools for Foster Parents, by Lana Temple-Plotz, Michael Sterba, and Ted P. Stricklett (Boys Town Press, 2002). From the good people of Boys and Girls Town, this is a real-world guide to issues big and small for foster parents, such as building attachment, relating to the foster child's parents, and handling transitions.

Websites, Mailing Lists, Blogs, and Social Media

Cancer and Fertility/Young People with Cancer

Planet Cancer (www.planetcancer.org)

This online gathering place for young adults with cancer has something for everyone: research updates, humor and "cancertainment," real-world advice, and wildly active forums, blogs, and affinity groups. PC strikes a welcome irreverent tone—their slogan is "We've done drugs Keith Richards never heard of." Their advocacy has helped to create young adult cancer support programs at many cancer centers across the country. In 2009,

Planet Cancer became an official program of the Lance Armstrong Foundation.

Crazy Sexy Life (www.crazysexylife.com)

A vibrant web community launched by "crazy sexy" cancer survivor Kris Carr, with blogs, forums, healthy recipes, and a newsletter, Crazy Sexy focuses on a holistic approach to cancer survivorship. The site's for all ages, but lots of young female survivors congregate here.

Breastcancer.org

One of the biggest online resources for breast cancer information, breastcancer.org has a wealth of information for women with breast cancer, including a special section of their popular message boards for younger women. They also have an excellent fertility, pregnancy, and adoption section at www.breastcancer .org/tips/fert_preg_adopt/, including the archives of a fascinating, in-depth ask-the-expert conference hosted in 2008. Check out the whole site at www.breastcancer.org.

TC-Cancer.com (www.tc-cancer.com)

This site offers support forums, blogs, treatment guides, personal stories, and the latest in research for the testicular cancer survivor.

Cancer and Careers (www.cancerandcareers.org)

Nothing here about fertility or parenting, but let's face it, most young cancer survivors are also juggling professional concerns while dealing with building a family. Cancer and Careers can help you manage paperwork with a huge virtual toolkit of checklists and charts, connect you with a career coach, and advise you on dealing with Human Resources and your boss.

Young Cancer Connection, Facebook

The MD Anderson Cancer Center organized this Facebook group to provide resources for young adults with cancer.

General Fertility

Fertile Thoughts

This is a huge online community of people dealing with fertility and infertility issues. Their popular forums have tens of thousands of members and include sections on cancer and infertility, and on premature ovarian failure. This is a great place to connect with others who have been down the same road. Find them at www.fertilethoughts.com.

Adoption and Fostering

Adoption-after-cancer

You might be surprised at just how active and busy the traffic is on this email listserv, which is aimed at people who've adopted after cancer or who are now in the process. If you want to keep your finger on the pulse of what adoption is like for cancer survivors right now—for example, if you want to talk to someone who's in the process of adopting from the same country you're considering—adoption-after-cancer is the place to go. Join the list here: groups.yahoo.com/group/adoption-after-cancer.

Adoption-agency-research

This mailing list is another must for prospective adoptive parents. Its official mission is to help prospective adoptive parents who are researching international adoption, but there's a lot of traffic about domestic adoption as well. This is the place to check out the agencies you're considering. Sign up at groups.yahoo.com/group/Adoption_Agency_Research.

Adoption.com

One of the biggest and most popular adoption-related sites on the Web, adoption.com has a busy, popular set of online forums as well as blogs and a lot of background information on adoption.

Adoptionvoices.com

This is an adoption social network with forums, blogs, affinity groups, and a chat area.

Creating a Family (www.creatingafamily.com)

I've categorized this one under adoption, but Dawn Davenport's amazing site covers a lot on both adoption and fertility issues. She hosts an excellent online radio show that frequently features some of the top experts in the field, and she maintains an outstanding set of fact sheets and resource listings on a huge array of topics in adoption and fertility, ranging from blending a family of adopted and biological children to embryo donation and sensory processing disorders. Dawn also writes a thought-provoking blog.

BeaFosterParent.com

This is a joint effort by foster care and adoption agencies in several states to reach out to potential foster parents. It guides you through the process and provides links to participating states and agencies.

Twitter Feeds

You can follow these twitter feeds, which are related to cancer, young survivors, fertility, adoption, and parenting:

@ASCO (the American Society for Clinical Oncology)

@BCsurvivors (gathering news about breast cancer survivors)

@CancerandCareers (the Cancer and Careers Foundation)

@conceive (*Conceive* magazine)

@cure_magazine

@DawnDavenport1 (Dawn Davenport of Creating a Family)

@fertilehopelnb (Lindsay Nohr Beck of Fertile Hope)

@hayeslat (Brandon Hayes-Lattin, an adolescent/young adult oncologist at Portland's Oregon Health Sciences University)

@heidisa (Heidi Adams, founder of Planet Cancer and director of grassroots engagement for Livestrong.com)

@Kairol (Kairol Rosenthal, author of *Everything Changes: The Insider's Guide to Cancer in Your 20s and 30s*)

@LanceArmstrong (you know this guy)

@LivestrongCEO (Doug Ulman, survivor and CEO of the Lance Armstrong Foundation)

@oncofertility (the Oncofertility Consortium)

@stop2ndguessing (Jen Singer, author of the *Stop 2nd Guessing Yourself* guides to parenting and the parenting-with-cancer host on Planet Cancer)

@stupidcancer (Matthew Zachary, survivor and founder of the I'm Too Young for This! Cancer Foundation)

@survivors (the Voices of Survivors Foundation)

@YSCBuzz (the Young Survival Coalition)

Magazines

Cancer and Fertility/Young People with Cancer

CURE

The best and only true feature and news magazine for people with all types of cancer, at all stages of the journey. There is a lot of material of interest to younger survivors and those of us trying to have children, like blogging from the Young Survival Coalition conference and a great feature on CML survivor and two-time mom Erin Zammett Ruddy. On their site, curetoday.com, you can search past articles by stage of the cancer journey, cancer type, and author name. The site also hosts blogs and message boards. Sign up online for a free subscription at www.curetoday.com or just read it online!

Mamm

The only magazine dedicated solely to the interests of women who've had breast or reproductive cancer, *Mamm* is for women of all ages but frequently devotes coverage to fertility and issues of interest to young survivors, like a recent article on "Sex and the Single Survivor." (One way you know you've found a man and not a boy, the article notes: "He finds you beautiful and sexy, and he loves to kiss your scars.") Subscribe by calling 877-668-1800 or look at online articles and archives at www.mamm.com.

General Fertility

Conceive

This is *the* magazine for men and women dealing with fertility issues. First published in 2004, the online version of the magazine now has a treasure trove of useful articles on everything from choosing an egg donor or sperm donor to which household cleaners could hurt your fertility. They're mostly about fertility/ infertility, but *Conceive* doesn't shortchange adoption either. The website also hosts blogs and personalized forums. Subscribe at www.conceiveonline.com.

Adoption

Adoptive Families

This is the biggest and most comprehensive adoption magazine out there. I've already talked plenty about all the resources *AF* offers on its website and in its books. If you're an adoptive parent or want to be one, you'll look forward eagerly to the day each new issue of *AF* arrives in your mailbox. Subscribe online at www .adoptivefamilies.com.

Adoption Today and Fostering Families Today

AT is the only magazine devoted entirely to international and transracial adoption, dealing with issues like race, schools, bonding, and choosing a country from which to adopt. *FFT* tackles everything from maintaining relationships with a birth family to dealing with sexualized behaviors in children. Subscribe to either or both online at www.adoptiontoday.com. These magazines are now all digital.

Notes

Introduction

1. Upponi, S., et al. Pregnancy after breast cancer. *European Journal of Cancer* (April 2003).

Chapter 1

1. Quinn, G. P., et al. Physician referral for fertility preservation in oncology patients: A national study of practice behaviors. *Journal of Clinical Oncology* 27, no. 35 (December 10, 2009): 5952–57.

2. Woodruff, T. In conversation with author. November 24, 2009.

3. Rueffer, U., et al. Male gonadal dysfunction in patients with Hodgkin's disease prior to treatment. *Annals of Oncology* 12, no. 9 (September 2001): 1307–11.

4. Jacobson, R., et al. Risk of testicular cancer in men with abnormal semen characteristics: Cohort study. *British Medical Journal* 321 (September 30, 2000): 789–92.

5. Oktay, K., et al. Association of BRCA1 mutations with occult primary ovarian insufficiency: A possible explanation for the link between infertility and breast/ovarian cancer risks. *Journal of Clinical Oncology* 28, no. 2 (January 10, 2010): 240–4.

6. Katz, D., et al. Fertility and pregnancy in patients under age 38 following chemotherapy for breast cancer. *Journal of Clinical Oncology* 27 (suppl; abstr; 2009): e11541.

7. Simon, B., et al. Preserving fertility after cancer. *CA: A Cancer Journal for Clinicians* 55 (2005): 211–28.

8. Fertile Hope. Fertility risks. www.fertilehope.org/learn-more/cancer-and-fertility-info/fertility-risks.cfm. (2010); Stearns, V., et al. Breast cancer treatment and ovarian failure: Risk factors and emerging genetic determinants. *Nature Reviews: Cancer* (November 6, 2006); Drugs@FDA. http://www.accessdata.fda.gov/scripts/cder/drugsatfda (manufacturer information for each drug).

9. Chung, K. In conversation with author. October 7, 2009.

10. Rovó, A., et al. Spermatogenesis in long-term survivors after allogeneic hematopoietic stem cell transplantation is associated with age, time interval since transplantation, and apparently absence of chronic GvHD. *Blood* 108, no. 3 (August 1, 2006): 1100–1105.

11. Lee, C. In conversation with author. September 30, 2009.

12. Sklar, C. A., et al. Premature menopause in survivors of childhood cancer: A report from the childhood cancer survivor study. *Journal of the National Cancer Institute* 98, no. 13 (July 5, 2006): 890–96.

13. Haukvik, U. K., et al. Treatment-related premature ovarian failure as a long-term complication after Hodgkin's lymphoma. *Annals of Oncology* 17, no. 9 (2006): 1428–33.

Chapter 2

1. Foster, R., and Bihrle, R. Current status of retroperitoneal lymph node dissection and testicular cancer: When to operate. *Cancer Control* 9, no. 4 (2002).

2. Baynosa, J., et al. Timing of breast cancer treatments with oocyte retrieval and embryo cryopreservation. *Journal of the American College of Surgeons* 209, no. 5 (November 2009): 603–7.

3. Azim, A., Constantini-Ferrando, M., and Oktay, K. Safety of fertility preservation by ovarian stimulation with letrozole and gonadotropins in patients with breast cancer: A prospective controlled study. *Journal of Clinical Oncology* 26, no. 16 (June 1, 2008): 2630–35.

4. Quinn, G. In conversation with author. October 20, 2009.

5. Krotz, S. P., et al. In vitro maturation of oocytes via the pre-fabricated self-assembled artificial human ovary. *Journal of Assisted Reproduction and Genetics* Epub ahead of print (August 25, 2010).

6. Gerrity, M. B. In conversation with author. November 24, 2009.

7. Dolmans, M. M., et al. Reimplantation of cryopreserved ovarian tissue from patients with acute lymphoblastic leukemia is potentially unsafe. *Blood* 116, no. 16 (October 21, 2010): 2908–14. Epub July 1, 2010.

8. Gonfloni, S., et al. Inhibition of the c-Abl-TAp63 pathway protects mouse oocytes from chemotherapy-induced death. *Nature Medicine* 15, no. 10 (October 2009): 1179–85. Epub September 27, 2009.

9. Provided courtesy of the Oncofertility Consortium. http:// oncofertility.northwestern.edu/health-professionals/ fertility-preservation-billing-resources.

Chapter 3

1. Therapeutic Sperm Banking. The Center for Reproductive Medicine, The Cleveland Clinic, Cleveland, Ohio. http://www.clevelandclinic .org/reproductiveresearchcenter/info/patientinfo2.html.

2. Beadle, B. M., et al. The impact of pregnancy on breast cancer outcomes in women ≤ 35 years. *Cancer* 115 (2009):1174–84.

Chapter 5

1. Cost of Adoption Update, 2008-2009. *Adoptive Families*. http://www.adoptivefamilies.com/articles.php?aid=2076.

2. Ibid.

Chapter 6

1. Oktay, K. In conversation with author. December 15, 2009.

2. Jacobson, H., et al. A proposed unified mechanism for the reduction of human breast cancer risk by the hormones of pregnancy. *Cancer Prevention Research* 3 (February 2010): 212.

3. Partridge, A. In conversation with author. January 12, 2010.

4. Marsh, K., Ormond, K., and Pergament, E. Cancer, chemotherapy and pregnancy. *Newsletter of the Illinois Teratogen Information Service* 7, no. 1 (October 1998).

5. Hilakivi-Clarke, L., et al. Maternal exposure to Tamoxifen during pregnancy increases carcinogen-induced mammary tumorigenesis among female rat offspring. *Clinical Cancer Research* 6, no. 1 (January 2000): 305; Possible Herceptin side effects. Genentech (manufacturer's labeling). http://www.herceptin.com/adjuvant/ breast-cancer-treatment/side-effects.jsp.

6. Serletti, J. Ask-the-Expert Online Conference: Reconstruction Updates. Breastcancer.org. May 2007. http://www.breastcancer.org/ treatment/surgery/reconstruction/ask_expert/2007_05/.

7. Weiss, M. Screening for breast cancer during pregnancy. Breastcancer .org. http://www.breastcancer.org/tips/fert_preg_adopt/bc_pregnancy/ screening.jsp.

8. Romine, L., Mattrey, R., and Brown, M. MR imaging of placenta accreta. Abstract presented to the Radiological Society of North America (RSNA) 95th Annual Meeting, December 2009.

9. Higgins, S., and Haffty, B. G. Pregnancy and lactation after breast-conserving therapy for early stage breast cancer. *Cancer* 73, no. 8 (April 15, 1994): 2175–80.

10. Stuebe, A., et al. Lactation and incidence of premenopausal breast cancer: A longitudinal study. *Archives of Internal Medicine* 169, no. 15 (2009): 1364–71.

Chapter 7

1. Rauch, P. In conversation with author. February 25, 2010.

About the Author

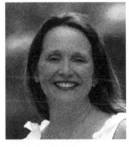 GINA M. SHAW is a health and medical writer and breast cancer survivor. She is also the mother of three children following her breast cancer diagnosis in 2004. Gina chronicled her journey through breast cancer in her thirties for *Redbook* in a five-part diary series. She has won awards for her medical feature writing, including the Society of Professional Journalists' award for a WebMD series, "Crossing the Thin Line," and the Association of Women in Communications' Clarion Award for another *Redbook* series, "The Fertility Diaries," which told the story of three Ohio women, their friendship, and their journey through fertility struggles, pregnancy, and parenthood. Her credits have also appeared in *Ladies' Home Journal, Fitness, Woman's Day,* and *WebMD the Magazine.*

Gina's daughter Annika was adopted in domestic open adoption in 2006, her son, Adrian, was born in March 2008 with no assisted reproduction, and her latest bundle of joy, Katia, arrived earlier this year. Along with husband Evan, they all live in Montclair, New Jersey.

Index